aromatherapy

in essence

aromatherapy

in essence

Nicola Jenkins

Hodder Arnold

A MEMBER OF THE HODDER HEADLINE GROUP

Orders: please contact Bookpoint Ltd, 130 Milton Park, Abingdon, Oxon OX14 4SB. Telephone: (44) 01235 827720. Fax: (44) 01235 400454. Lines are open from 9.00 – 5.00, Monday to Saturday, with a 24 hour message answering service. You can also order through our website www.hoddereducation.co.uk

If you have any comments to make about this, or any of our other titles, please send them to educationenquiries@hodder.co.uk

British Library Cataloguing in Publication Data
A catalogue record for this title is available from the British Library

ISBN-10: 0 340 92606 6
ISBN-13: 978 0 340 92606 2

This Edition Published 2006
Impression number   10 9 8 7 6 5 4 3 2 1
Year   2010 2009 2008 2007 2006

Hodder Headline's policy is to use papers that are natural, renewable and recyclable products and made from wood grown in sustainable forests. The logging and manufacturing processes are expected to conform to the environmental regulations of the country of origin.

The information given in this book is not intended as a replacement for medical advice and should not be used for diagnosis or treatment of any medical condition.

Cover photo from Simon Watson/Taxi/Getty Images
Artwork by Oxford Designers and Illustrators

Printed and bound in Great Britain for Hodder Arnold, an imprint of Hodder Education, a member of the Hodder Headline Group, 338 Euston Road, London NW1 3BH by CPI Bath

contents

acknowledgements

This book would have been far more difficult to write if it hadn't been for the support, advice, and encouragement of a number of key people. Thanks are especially due to Deike Begg and to Anne Gamble. I'd also like to thank Jennie Harding for the moisturising gel recipe quoted on page 46; Sophie Darragh for babysitting at short notice; Lesley Bacon, Susan Yadlon and Annette Van for their support and encouragement and my current and former students for their willingness to donate their bodies to science as they tried out blends and asked a lot of complicated questions in the process. You have all helped me to hone my ideas and keep the explanations (relatively) simple. Lastly, this is, as always, for Alan and Hannah.

The author and publishers would like to thank the following for the use of photographs in this volume:

p. 3 Cordelia Molloy/Science Photo Library, p. 5 akg-images, p. 9 Nick Spurling/Holt/FLPA, p. 30 (left) Keith Rushford/FLPA (right) Tim Fitzharris/FLPA, p. 31 (left) Martin B Withers/FLPA (right) WoodyStock/Alamy, p. 32 (left) Roger Cope/Holt/FLPA (top right) Fred Hazelhoff/Foto Natura/FLPA (bottom right) Bob Gibbons/Holt/FLPA, p. 33 (left) Nigel Cattlin/Holt/FLPA (right) Jurgen & Christine Sohns/FLPA, p. 34 (left) © Gunter Rossenbach/Zefa/Corbis (right) Nigel Cattlin/Holt/FLPA, p. 35 (top left) P. Karanukaran/Holt/FLPA (bottom left) Jurgen & Christine Sohns/FLPA (right) © Michael Freeman/Corbis, p. 36 (left) Alan and Linda Detrick/Holt/FLPA (top right) Pascal Goetgheluck/Science Photo Library (bottom right) Arco Images/Alamy, p. 37 (left and right) P. Karanukaran/Holt/FLPA, p. 66 (top) © Paul Vozdic/Getty Images (bottom) © Matthias Clamer/Getty Images, p. 67 PurestockX, p. 68 (left) Hercules Robinson/Alamy (right), p. 78, p. 102, p. 116 Dr P. Marazzi/Science Photo Library, p. 87 Mark Douet/Getty Images, p. 118 Dr Najeeb Layyous/Sciemce Photo Library, p. 125 Lauren Shear/Science Photo Library

Commissioned photographs by Carl Drury.

With thanks to Minna and Stuart, our models, and to Images Model Agency.

Understanding aromatherapy

'. . . a rose, by any other name would smell as sweet.'

(William Shakespeare, *Romeo and Juliet*)

Fragrance has fascinated us for centuries; one brief hint of something in the air can transport us through time and space and it can ease the heart and the mind (or the lungs). But can it really help to heal? Those who practise aromatherapy would argue 'yes'. Here's why.

introducing
aromatherapy

Once upon a time, perhaps not very long ago, you picked up a bottle of essential oil for the first time. Perhaps it was a gift – chances are, it was lavender, or possibly tea tree. It might have come with some brief instructions for use: 'put it in a burner/in the bath/in some oil' and 'it's good for sleep, burns, or pain relief'. If it was the tea tree, perhaps it was suggested for athlete's foot, as an antiseptic, or as a polite reminder that your trainers were a little too fragrant.

That was when you got hooked.

More than any other complementary therapy, aromatherapy has the ability to inspire clients and practitioners alike, because it offers the chance to create a completely personal response to any health issues. It nurtures from the inside out. Even if you have no desire to practise aromatherapy massage, you can benefit from the treatment and create a personal response to whatever issues you are

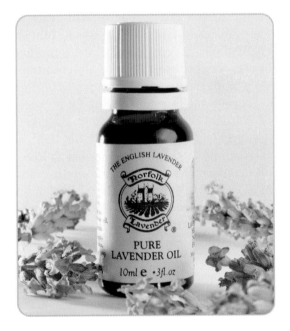

facing. All you need is a choice of essential oils, an idea of what to do with them and the urge to express yourself in fragrance.

The power of aromatherapy

Our sense of smell is arguably the most evocative sense we have. As you may have heard, estate agents sometimes suggest that vendors brew fresh coffee before a visit from prospective buyers in order to encourage them to feel at home. In some parts of the world, department stores use essential oils to encourage customers to relax and to buy more products. Hospices and nursing homes have experimented with vaporising lavender (in particular) in order to encourage better quality sleep and a feeling of well-being in their patients. Many baby products contain essential oils (at very low doses) to improve health, well-being and, above all, encourage sleep in the smallest people among us.

People come to aromatherapy for a variety of reasons. Some try it because they love massage and think that the addition of essential oils to the massage oil may enhance the treatment, making it more effective and more enjoyable. Others love the essential oils: a fragrance they encounter in a bath product or in a candle gets them hooked, possibly with a desire to create and make their own products. Others try it because they are looking for a change of pace, a deeper sense of meaning in their lives, or just time to be themselves without worrying about anyone else's needs. Whatever it is they are searching for, aromatherapy tends to inspire, not least for its combination of opportunities to nurture yourself and others, to create and to play.

A look at the history

There is some discussion over when aromatherapy was first developed. It could be said that it originated in the 1960s when the Austrian biochemist, Marguerite Maury, first wrote *The Secrets of Life and Youth*, in which she established the use of essential oils in cosmetics and massage; and that it was consolidated over a decade later, in 1977, when Robert Tisserand wrote *The Art of Aromatherapy*, the first book on the subject written in the English language.

However, there is a far richer and more complex background to the use of essential oils for therapeutic, medicinal and culinary use. It is from the traditional and ancient uses of essential oils that today's therapists derive knowledge of some of the properties that are ascribed to the individual oils. When biomedical research is carried out, it often confirms the properties already known by users of essential oils through the ages.

Key moments in aromatherapy's history

2000 BCE:	Medicinal properties of black pepper noted in Chinese and Sanskrit texts
1500 BCE:	Egyptians using cedarwood, frankincense, cypress and myrrh for embalming, cosmetics and perfumery
776 BCE:	Greece using essential oils in water for fragrances and as a specific distillation and incense to enhance prophetic abilities of the Oracles
496 BCE:	Kings of Persia and Babylon noted as receiving frankincense as tribute and pricing it weight for weight at the same value as gold
400 BCE:	Hippocrates recommending chamomile to reduce fever

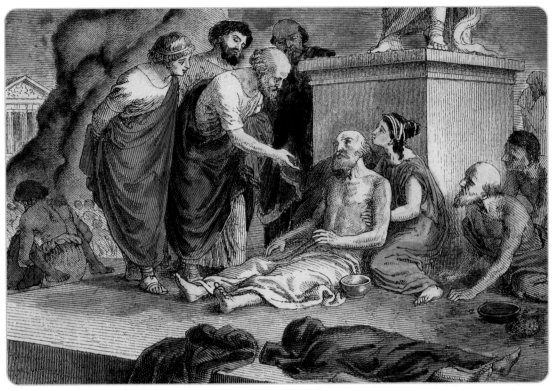

This woodcut depicts Hippocrates helping an ill man during the plague

165 CE:	Galen using cypress to relieve diarrhoea
500–600 CE:	Evidence in India of sandalwood being used for exorcism rites as well as for healing wounds
1000 CE:	Imports to China of frankincense destined for medical use
1030 CE:	Avicenna distilling roses both for the essential oil and for the hydrolat
1400 CE:	Friar's Balsam (frankincense and benzoin) used for respiratory and skin complaints
1550 CE:	Sandalwood used to treat cholera in China
1600 CE:	Bergamot used in Italian folk medicine
1649 CE:	Culpeper's text on herbal medicine published
1700 CE:	Eau de Cologne developed and goes into popular use
1850 CE:	Neroli used in bridal headdresses in England to symbolise purity
1875 CE:	Juniper berries burned to prevent smallpox from spreading in French hospitals
1910 CE:	French chemist Gattefosse burns his hand in his laboratory, sticks it in a vat of lavender essential oil and escapes with no lasting damage or pain – discovering in the process proof of lavender's effective use in pain and damage control for burns
1948–49 CE:	Dr Jean Valnet uses essential oils to treat battle wounds during the Indochina war.

In today's search for definitive answers, research into the effectiveness of essential oils for various conditions or circumstances continues to unearth interesting facts. Some fairly recent findings include:

- In a study carried out into the treatment of alopecia (where hair falls out in patches), those treated with a blend containing Atlas cedarwood showed significant improvement (44 per cent) in the hair's regrowth.[1]

- Clary sage, when used in labour, was shown to provide significant pain relief, relax the mother and to accelerate labour.[2]

- Although highly regarded for its antiseptic and antimicrobial activities, lemon also helps to stimulate the nervous system: studies carried out in Japan showed that when lemon was vaporised through a room, typing errors were reduced by 54 per cent. [3]

- Both palmarosa and lemongrass have been shown to offer almost complete protection against malaria-carrying mosquitoes for up to 11 hours.[4]

This book concentrates on giving you the information you need to use essential oils safely, creatively and effectively.

If your intention is to work as an aromatherapist, see the section 'Where to go from here' near the end of the book, for details on how to find a course to suit your needs and interests.

References

1 Hay, I.C., Jamieson, M., Ormerod, A.D. (1998) 'Randomized trial of aromatherapy: Successful treatment of alopecia areata', Arch Dermatol

2 Burns, E., Blamey, C, 'Soothing scents in childbirth', The International Journal of Aromatherapy, 6(1): 24–28

3 Tisserand, R. (1988) 'Lemon fragrance increases office efficiency', The International Journal of Aromatherapy 1988, 1(2)

4 Ansari, M. A., Razdan, R.K. 'Relative efficacy of various oils in repelling mosquitoes', Indian J Malariol, 32(3): 104–11. Cited in the Aromatherapy Database, Bob Harris Essential Oil Consultants, UK 2000.

Note: These studies (and many more) are all quoted in *The Complete Guide to Aromatherapy*, by Salvatore Battaglia (2004), one of the most comprehensive textbooks for aromatherapy at practitioner and undergraduate level and above.

the science
behind aromatherapy

First and foremost, aromatherapy is a holistic therapy. This means that practitioners take into consideration the physical, mental, spiritual, emotional and environmental needs of clients when making decisions about how treatments will be carried out. The enormous variety of essential oils available and the methods of applying them encourage a holistic approach. You could have several people before you who all have headaches arising from a similar condition, but the appropriate treatment will vary from person to person, depending on your assessment of their circumstances. There will be several options about how to proceed.

The range of treatment options available can leave aromatherapy open to dispute, with some people questioning just how effective it really is. Standard methods of experimentation insist that you need to be able to replicate both the results and experimental procedures in order to state definitively that any findings are valid. So, for example, all batches of a particular essential oil would need to consist of the same levels of chemical constituents. Also, all the people or animals used as subjects to test reactions to the particular oil would need to respond in the same way. Therein lies the problem: different batches of the same type of oil vary, as do individual responses to them.

Why essential oils vary

While there is an increasing number of research projects testing the effectiveness of aromatherapy and of individual essential oils, it is very difficult to get two batches of essential oils that are exactly the same, even if they are harvested from the same area. The potency, fragrance and chemical makeup of any essential oil will vary according to the following criteria:

- soil type
- climate – especially if there is unseasonable weather
- use of pesticides – organic fertilisers and pesticides can affect the final product
- amount of water available as the plant is growing (both drought and too much rain can be problematic)
- time of harvest (and whether the plant has had enough time to develop, especially if the weather has been bad). This is a particular problem with some of the species grown in areas where harvesting is not always appropriately regulated – for example, where rosewood is harvested in the South American rainforests, or sandalwood in India. As the trees become scarce, younger trees are being harvested and not always replaced. As well as lowering the quality of the essential oil, the effect on the environment and local habitats is undesirable
- altitude – the same variety, grown at different altitudes, will have a markedly different fragrance and potency.

As a result, many of the essential oil growers and suppliers commission complex tests (usually, one of these is gas liquid chromatography) to identify the percentage at which each chemical constituent is present in the essential oil. The tests consititute one of the methods used for ensuring that the quality and effectiveness of the essential oil meets certain standards. Most reputable essential oil suppliers list the batch number on the bottle of essential oil so that they can easily identify where the contents came from and, if necessary, refer to records of the quality testing if customers have any questions about it.

Maintaining the quality and effectiveness of your essential oils

Once you have purchased your essential oils, it is important to make sure that they stay fresh for as long as possible. Storing them properly can help to increase their shelf life:

- Keep them out of direct sunlight. The oils will usually be sold to you in dark bottles, but also try to keep them out of the light as much as possible.
- Keep them at a stable temperature – the colder the better. Many therapists store their essential oils in the fridge, although this isn't always necessary, as long as they are not prone to sudden or extreme changes in temperature. (Storing them in the bathroom, for example, is not a good idea.)
- Ensure that lids are properly replaced. Essential oils start to oxidise once they are in contact with the air. You can prevent this from happening by replacing lids as quickly as possible.
- Buy essential oils in small quantities. They all have a recommended shelf life. Most are sold in 10 ml containers (although you can buy expensive essential oils such as rose, neroli or jasmine in 2.5 and 5 ml quantities).

Check the shelf life. Many suppliers list the expected shelf life on individual bottles. Most essential oils last for about two years after purchase. Citrus oils last for about six months. Storing them appropriately can extend the shelf life.

Try this:

Compare lavender oils grown in different circumstances to see if you can smell the differences between them. For example, you may want to compare French and English or Italian lavenders; or perhaps a variety that was organically grown with its non-organic counterpart; or a high-altitude lavender with one that was grown at lower altitude. Think about how they make you feel – do some have a more sedative effect than the others?

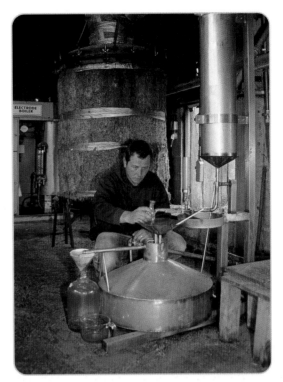
A lavender still

Harvesting essential oils

Essential oils are extracted from their sources by one of four different methods, according to the nature of the plant product (whether it is a herb, a fruit, a flower or a tree) and the amount of essential oil it yields. The four main methods of extraction are:

1 Distillation. This is the most common method of extraction. Using either water or steam, large amounts of plant material are heated under pressure and the molecules of steam and essential oil are then condensed (so that they return from gas to liquid form) and collected. The essential oil floats on top of the condensation product. The hydrolat remains behind.

2 Enfleurage. This is one method of extracting essential oils from exotic flowers. The flowers are placed in oil and left in the sunlight for an extended length of time so that the essential oils will be gently released. After a while, the oil is strained and the flowers replaced until the essential oil is present at the required level. Alcohol is then used to get the essential oil out of the base oil.

3 Expression. This is used to harvest citrus oils (the essential oil is found in the peel of the citrus fruit – you use it every time you scrape the zest of an orange or lemon when cooking). The peel is squeezed in a variety of methods in order to extract the essential oil without heating or damaging it in any way.

aromatherapy in essence

4 Solvent extraction. This is used to extract essential oils that would be degraded beyond use if they were distilled. Usually, the extraction process requires either alcohol or another strong chemical, although increasingly carbon dioxide is used for this process as it can be removed more easily from the end product.

How the essential oils enter the body

Just as plants and essential oils are subject to variation in quality and effectiveness, the way in which they enter the human body, and our responses to them once they get there, also varies. There are three key ways that the essential oils used in aromatherapy get into the body:

- via the skin
- via the sense of smell (olfaction)
- via the lungs.

The skin

The most common way of using aromatherapy is to apply essential oils as part of a massage. The essential oils are mixed with a vegetable carrier oil, into which they dissolve. This blend is then applied to the skin. The structure of the carrier oil and of the essential oils makes it possible for the essential oils to be absorbed into the skin. From there, they can enter the underlying tissues, affecting the nerves, the blood stream and the other organs of the body. You can increase the rate at which the essential oils are absorbed – for example, by heating the area after you have applied the massage blend. This could be done using a hot water bottle or

Try this:

Essential oils really can enter the body via the skin. Prove it to yourself using garlic essential oil. Cut a clove of garlic in half and rub the liquid that emerges from the clove on the base of your foot. Note how long it takes before you can taste garlic on your breath. (It usually takes about 20 minutes.)

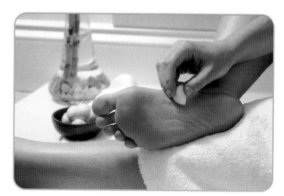

The garlic test

a heated wheat bag, or by covering the area with towels or blankets.

The sense of smell (olfaction)

Deep within the nasal passage lie the receptors for smell. These nerve endings, called chemoreceptors, respond to chemicals in solution. Airborne fragrance chemicals are dissolved in the fluids that coat the nasal membranes so that the nerve endings can respond to them and transport the 'chemical message' to the brain, indicating what smell is being experienced. The chemoreceptors are very unusual nerve cells in that they are continuously being renewed throughout adult life; usually they last only 60 days.

Studies carried out in the 1990s into how our sense of smell works showed that while there are no clear ways in which smells can be identified and classified (which is why aromatherapists tend to use the vocabulary supplied by the perfume industry to describe the fragrance of an essential oil), the research was able show that the receptors were stimulated by different combinations of smells and that, as well as responding to pleasant fragrances, the chemoreceptors also respond to smells they identify as painful – noticeably, menthol, chilli and ammonia. Individuals learn how to identify the different combinations of smells and this ability can be developed and enhanced. (It is a natural development, as students of aromatherapy experience.)

Once a fragrant message is picked up by the olfactory nerve, it goes to two destinations within the brain. First, it goes via the thalamus to the frontal lobe of the brain. In this area, smells are consciously interpreted and analysed (this is the part of your brain that you are using when you do a smell test on an essential oil to analyse how it changes over time). The second route the fragrant message takes is via the hypothalamus and limbic system to the autonomic nervous system, where an emotional response to the fragrance is developed and where the truly visceral responses to an essential oil arise (including choking, sneezing, feeling endangered, feeling safe or sleepy, or feeling that the fragrance is transporting you back to another time or experience). Perhaps, for example, benzoin's vanilla-like fragrance takes you back to times when as a child, you baked cakes with your mother.

Via the lungs

The lungs are the most effective excretory organ in the body, getting rid of approximately 60 per cent of all our waste products. The same features that make the lungs so effective at excretion also make them effective at absorbing oxygen (as you breathe in) and essential oils as they are vaporised. Once gaseous molecules of essential oil are inhaled they enter the alveoli, the smallest chambers of the lungs. These tiny chambers are separated from the surrounding capillaries by a single-celled wall, allowing blood and air to come into very close contact, so that diffusion of oxygen (going into the blood) and carbon dioxide (coming out of the blood) is possible. Inhaling the fragrance of essential oils therefore allows them to enter your bloodstream very quickly and start to work.

What essential oils can do

Essential oils have been attributed with a number of properties, most of which are based either on traditional uses or are currently or recently under investigation. Their effectiveness at each activity varies according to the essential oil. Some of these properties are shown in the table on page 13.

While the ability of essential oils to bring about physical changes has been noticed and is subject to frequent testing, there has been some doubt about how essential oils affect the mind and nervous system. We know they *do* work – for example, the use of lavender as a sedative is well documented. One possibility is that once the essential oils enter the body they

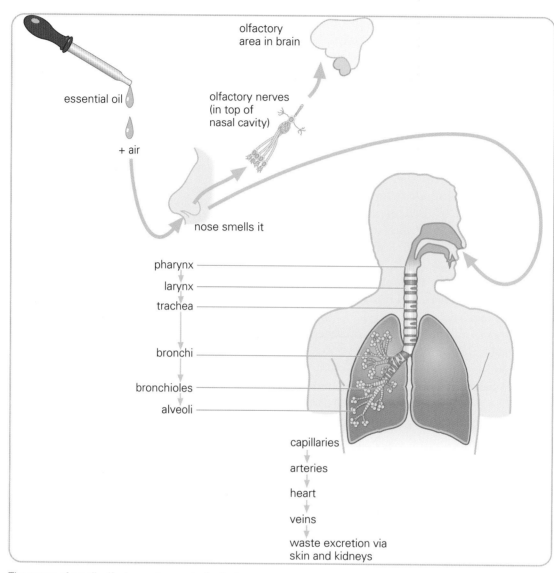

The sense of smell: olfactory pathways to the brain

can (and do) act in a similar way to specific *neurotransmitters* – chemicals involved in the response the nerves make to changes within the body. By using essential oils that mimic certain neurotransmitters, we are trying to increase the feel-good effects of those neurotransmitters, and help someone over an emotional 'blip' they may be experiencing.

Neurotransmitters are very interesting substances; a small amount can make us feel so euphoric, yet when an imbalance occurs – such as when someone falls into depression – it can take a long time to help them back to a state of balance. Anti-depressants, for instance, are usually prescribed with a view to someone staying on them for at least three months (six is often preferable) and that while they are on

What the essential oils appear to do when they get into the body

Characteristic	Definition	Exemplar essential oils
Analgesic	Painkillers that can mimic neurotransmitters and interfere with the pain signals sent out by the body.	Peppermint, lemongrass, clove, rosemary.
Antibiotic	Kills bacteria.	Tea tree, lavender.
Antifungal	Kills fungal infections.	Tea tree, lemongrass, manuka.
Anti-inflammatory	Reduces inflammation.	Yarrow, German chamomile, lavender, clove.
Antiseptic	Kills bacteria (for use on the skin).	Tea tree, lavender, manuka.
Antispasmodic	Stops muscle spasms.	Marjoram, rosemary, peppermint, cedarwood.
Antiviral	Kills viruses.	Melissa, tea tree, lavender, lemon
Aphrodisiac	Encourages sexual interest.	Black pepper, jasmine, rose, sandalwood.
Astringent	Dries up mucus, dries up other secretions (including sebum in the skin), slows bleeding.	Cypress, frankincense, sandalwood.
Carminative	Soothes and settles the digestive system, easing any stomach cramps, reduces flatulence and ensures that peristalsis (the wave-like contractions that move food through the gastro-intestinal tract) is regular and effective.	Peppermint, fennel, chamomile, melissa.
Cytophylactic	Encourages the healthy and appropriate growth of skin and other tissues.	Lavender, cedarwood, frankincense.
Diuretic	Increases urine production and helps reduce water retention	Juniper, grapefruit, lemon.
Euphoric	Improves mood. Some actively mimic neurotransmitters that reduce anxiety and depression too.	Neroli, Roman chamomile, jasmine, orange, grapefruit, rose.
Emmenagogue	Brings on menstruation.	Rose, geranium, basil, clary sage, chamomile, rosemary, ginger, marjoram, juniper.
Expectorant	Encourages the removal of mucus and catarrh from the lungs and sinuses.	Eucalyptus, fennel, rosemary, cypress, sandalwood, cedarwood, pine, clary sage.

Characteristic	Definition	Exemplar essential oils
Hormonal (generally)	Balances hormone production and dispersal. Some essential oils are structurally similar to specific hormones and can mimic their effects in the body. Other essential oils can help to improve blood flow (hormones are transported via the blood).	Jasmine, clary sage and fennel, geranium, rose, neroli.
Laxative	Clears congestion in the bowels.	Peppermint, black pepper, marjoram, fennel, orange, pine.
Rubefacient	Causes reddening of the skin (improves circulation).	Rosemary, peppermint, black pepper, lemongrass.
Sedative	Induces sleep; the aroma can encourage you to feel safe and able to rest, and can affect your sleep/wake cycle, encouraging you to rest effectively.	Lavender, Roman chamomile, German chamomile, carrot seed, vetiver, valerian.
Sudorific	Encourages sweating.	Basil, cardamom, ginger, rosemary, black pepper.
Vasoconstrictor	Causes the walls of the blood vessels to contract.	Cypress.
Vasodilator	Causes the walls of the blood vessels to relax.	Black pepper, eucalyptus, marjoram, rosemary.
Vulnerary	Heals wounds.	Lavender, frankincense.

the treatment they are addressing whatever emotional or physical issues triggered the condition in the first place.

Equally, if someone is trying to overcome an addiction, results do not happen overnight. When a substance such as nicotine or, more seriously, cocaine or heroin, is introduced to the body, it produces a very strong reaction, which the body perceives as the supply of a particular neurotransmitter from an outside source. Because it is getting the neurotransmitter from elsewhere, it sometimes ceases to manufacture it, which then induces cravings for the substance at ever increasing levels. Part of overcoming addiction is for the body to start producing the neurotransmitter the drug was mimicking at the required levels for that person to function normally.

Neurotransmitters simplified

Neurotransmitter	Action	Potential problems
Acetyl choline	Stimulates muscles to contract.	Release inhibited by botulinum (the substance used in botox treatments for the face); too little found in some areas of the brain in Alzheimer's sufferers; linked to a smoker's response to nicotine.
Noradrenalin	Energises the individual; involved in the emotions; regulates biological clock.	Cocaine mimics this, as do certain anti-depressants.
Dopamine	The feel-good neurotransmitter; involved in the emotions; regulates biological clock.	Too much leads to schizophrenia; too little is linked to Parkinsons. Reuptake is blocked by cocaine (so someone feels low after the cocaine starts to wear off).
Serotonin	Involved in sleep, appetite, nausea, migraine, and regulation of mood.	Too little leads to depression. The SSRI group of anti-depressants (such as Prozac) block its reuptake in order to relieve anxiety and depression.
Endorphins	Reduces perception of pain.	Inhibits pain.
Enkephalins	Reduces perception of pain.	Inhibits pain.

the science behind aromatherapy

FAQs – About the science behind aromatherapy

Why is it important to know about the chemical constituents of the essential oils?

It isn't important unless you are going to become a professional aromatherapist. Knowing about the chemical constituents helps therapists to make decisions about which blends of essential oils are going to be more effective for their client and which essential oils a client might have an adverse reaction to and why. Knowing the chemical constituents also allows the professional therapist to ensure that they don't blend essential oils with similar chemical constituents together in such a way that the client would be exposed to dangerously high concentrations of a particular chemical.

Why is it that after a while, I don't notice the smell of my perfume anymore?

One of the special adaptations of the olfactory nerve cells is that they have accessory (helper) cells called mitral cells, which help to refine the nerve signal (in this case, the concentration of the perfume's fragrance), amplify it and then relay it to the brain. These mitral cells also produce a specific chemical, which inhibits all but the strongest messages from being sent. It is believed that this inhibiting action is involved in what they call olfactory adaptation, where you stop noticing a particular fragrance. However, this doesn't mean that everyone around you can't smell your perfume!

I've lost my sense of smell, can aromatherapy still benefit me?

The most common reasons why someone might lose their sense of smell include a head injury, inflammation in the nasal cavities (usually as a result of an allergy, a head cold or from smoking), obstruction of the nasal cavities or sinuses (usually polyps) and as a result of age. Zinc deficiency is also linked to the loss of the sense of smell. If you have lost your sense of smell, aromatherapy can still be of benefit to you because the essential oils will get into your skin and into your circulation. If you think that your sense of smell could return, try using inhalations of cardamom, lemon, or cypress (to clear the nasal cavities, reduce inflammation and reduce mucus production).

safety issues and contraindications

As distillations of plant extracts, essential oils need to be treated with care and consideration. In a 5 ml bottle of rose otto essential oil, for example, you have the product of around 500,000 roses, which in part accounts for the cost of this particularly valuable and sought-after product. Because essential oils are so concentrated, there are specific safety issues that must be taken into consideration.

Safety considerations checklist

- Do not take essential oils by mouth.
- Always dilute essential oils in a carrier oil – especially if you are applying them to the skin.
- Keep essential oils away from your eyes.
- Store essential oils out of the reach of children.
- Check for allergies to essential oils or carrier products by patch testing.
- See your doctor immediately if you react to any products.
- Recognise your personal limits – if in doubt about how to use aromatherapy safely or effectively (especially if it is a serious condition that you want to deal with), see a professional aromatherapist.
- Some medications increase the effectiveness of essential oils. If you are on medication, speak to a professional aromatherapist before using essential oils yourself.
- Never apply essential oils to broken skin or open wounds.
- Avoid sunbathing or using a sunbed after applying citrus essential oils, as they increase the skin's sensitivity to sunlight.

Patch testing

When you suspect that you might be sensitive to a particular essential oil or carrier product, it is safest to carry out a patch test in advance of treatment. For this, you need to apply two drops of the essential oil, undiluted, to a plaster. Place the plaster on the inside of your forearm and check your response over the next 24 hours. If there is no response, you are safe to proceed.

Special cases

The following physical conditions make using specific essential oils a dangerous prospect:

- Allergies – be particularly careful about the carrier oils that are linked to foods that often cause intolerance: wheatgerm, avocado, peanut, or sweet almond oils can occasionally cause an adverse reaction. Citrus allergies appear to be more common today. These would rule out using some (but not necessarily all) of the following essential oils: lemon, bergamot, orange, tangerine, lime, mandarin, neroli and petitgrain.

- Blood pressure – avoid rosemary, peppermint, hyssop and eucalyptus in cases of high blood pressure; avoid ylang ylang where there is low blood pressure.

- Asthma – avoid eucalyptus.

- Liver disease – avoid parsley seed and bay.

- Kidney disease – avoid parsley seed.

- Fever – avoid hyssop, rosemary, yarrow, and all varieties of lavender (apart from *Lavandula angustifolia*).

- Do not use the following essential oils neat in the bath or in an inhalation, as they will irritate sensitive mucus membranes and can also irritate the skin – basil, fennel, lemongrass, lemon, melissa, clove, oregano, thyme, bay, cinnamon, peppermint.

- These essential oils are best avoided or used in small doses if you suspect the skin is sensitive – clove, eucalyptus, lemongrass, may chang, melissa, oregano, thyme.

- These oils are classed as photosensitising – which means that it is best to avoid exposing the skin to sunlight or to a sunbed for at least 12 hours after applying them – angelica, bergamot, lemon, lime.

- Homeopathy – if you are receiving homeopathic medication, consult your homeopath. Some essential oils are contraindicated in homeopathic treatment – those that are most likely to be a problem include rosemary, tea tree, eucalyptus, bay, cinnamon and peppermint.

- Pregnancy and breastfeeding – the skin is more sensitive and porous at this time, and the essential oils can affect the foetus too. Avoid using essential oils on the skin during the first trimester of a pregnancy, especially where there is a history of miscarriage. After the first trimester, keep any blends down at one per cent, or less (four drops in 20 mls) and avoid using essential oils such as rosemary and tea tree. See Chapter 16 for suggestions of oils that are recommended for use in pregnancy.

- Infants under two years – use a maximum of two drops in 100 ml of carrier oil. Only use the essential oils recommended for use during pregnancy. If your child has sensitive skin, then it is wise to refrain from using all essential oils except lavender, Roman chamomile and tangerine or mandarin.

- Children under 12 years – use a maximum of one per cent essential oils in solution, or four drops in 20 mls.

- Healthy adults – use a maximum of two per cent essential oils in a carrier oil or product (eight drops in 20 ml of carrier oil).

- If you are working only on the face, my preference is to reduce this further to one per cent (four drops in 20 ml) only, as the skin on the face is more sensitive. (So on a pregnant woman, I reduce the dosage to 0.5 per cent in solution for the face, or two drops in 20 ml.)

Contraindications to aromatherapy

The word 'contraindication' refers to those situations where it is not appropriate to treat someone, i.e. treatment is contraindicated. Caution is required in other situations, perhaps with amendments to your usual practice. Some of the contraindications and cautions in aromatherapy are the same as you would expect in massage.

In the table on the following pages, 'total' means avoid treatment altogether; 'local' means you can work elsewhere on the body but not in the local area of the condition; and 'medical' indicates that permission to treat is required from the subject's GP or specialist.

Where contraindications are concerned, the general rule is that when you are uncertain it is best to avoid doing a treatment and suggest to the person that they visit their doctor for clarification. It is also important to recognise when you are out of your depth and refer the client on to another practitioner. Do not allow yourself to worsen a condition by acting in well-meaning ignorance.

Adverse reactions to aromatherapy

Occasionally, someone might react to the essential oils or the blend you have used. Usually, you will see the reaction on the skin.

Photosensitisation

This is commonly associated with the citrus essential oils. Some can increase the skin's ability to absorb ultraviolet light. The essential oils themselves are not phototoxic; however, it is specific chemical constituents that are found in the essential oil when it has been expressed, rather than distilled, that can cause this reaction. Of the citrus essential oils that are easily available, bergamot and lime are the most likely to cause photosensitisation. Orange, lemon, grapefruit, tangerine and mandarin have the same chemical constituents, but as they are used in smaller amounts they are much less likely to cause a reaction.

19

Contraindications to aromatherapy

Contraindication or caution	Condition	Reason to avoid treatment
Total	Any contagious or infectious skin condition	You could pick it up or pass it on. (However, you could consider making a moisturiser or body oil that contains essential oils to reduce any itchiness and help the person recover more quickly.)
Total	Severe, widespread psoriasis, eczema or dermatitis	Skin is more vulnerable in a flare-up, making sensitisation likely. Avoid oakmoss essential oil (this is a popular addition to some perfumes, mostly for men) in particular, but some essential oils, such as lavender, German chamomile, yarrow and cedarwood can be beneficial if applied as a moisturiser.
Total	Epilepsy	Some essential oils have been known to trigger an attack. Essential oils you should use with caution (or avoid) if you are epileptic include rosemary, peppermint, yarrow, fennel, hyssop and some varieties of lavender. Others have been used to prevent attacks (e.g. ylang ylang).
Total	Untreated severe medical problems	You could make things worse, or hide key symptoms.
Total	Pregnancy during the first 16 weeks	Risk of miscarriage. Some essential oils could be used in the inhalation method to relieve morning sickness, but avoid using them on the skin.
Total	Any conditions being treated by a doctor or medical specialist without their written approval	Use of essential oils could alter absorption and effectiveness of any medication. For example, if you are taking anticoagulants like aspirin, heparin or warfarin, you should avoid using bay, cinnamon or clove (among others). Aromatherapy massage will also increase the transdermal penetration of substances absorbed via patches placed on the skin – such as nicotine patches for those giving up smoking, or HRT patches.
Total	When under the influence of alcohol or recreational drugs	Increased side effects (including a more severe hangover). For example, clary sage is likely to result in a severe hangover if alcohol is taken before or just after having an aromatherapy massage.

Contraindication or caution	Condition	Reason to avoid treatment
Local	Bruises	Increased pain and associated internal bleeding. However, a cold compress with ginger could be used to ease the pain and reduce the appearance of the bruise.
Local	Cuts, grazes, stings, insect bites	Risk of infection.
Local	First three days of menstruation	Deep abdominal massage contraindicated as it can increase menstrual blood flow.
Local	During pregnancy	Deep abdominal massage to be avoided as it can be uncomfortable for mother and baby. Avoid these essential oils throughout pregnancy – hyssop, parsley seed, basil. Reduce the dilution of essential oils down to one per cent in solution.
Local	Immediately after a meal	Interferes with digestion and absorption of food
Local	Diarrhoea	Worsens cramping of abdominal muscles, accidents can happen.
Local	Varicose veins	Very light treatment can occasionally (in mild cases) be beneficial. Heavier treatments to be avoided.
Local	Recent scar tissue	In case scar opens up or bleeds, or underlying tissues have not yet healed.
Local	Over areas of inflammation, swelling or pain	These will be painful to touch. If they are inflamed for no apparent reason, seek medical advice.
Medical – permission to treat is required from the GP or specialist.	Diabetes	Okay to treat if clients monitor their blood sugar levels closely and regularly. Watch for the physiological changes that diabetics are prone to – loss of sensation in peripheral area, dry or damaged skin, slow wound healing, poor circulation, frequent bacterial and fungal infections (such as thrush or athlete's foot).
Medical	Heart conditions	Treatment affects blood pressure and blood flow, which could in turn affect the heart action.
Medical	On medication	Seek doctor's permission, as essential oils could interfere with medication prescribed.
Medical	Cancer	Possibility that cancer could spread as a result of massage (although there isn't much evidence of this). Get written permission.

Contraindication or caution	Condition	Reason to avoid treatment
Medical	Post-operative	Do not treat someone who is currently recovering from an operation without the doctor's written permission.
Medical	Severe swelling	Reason for the swelling needs to be identified and dealt with by a medical professional first before you consider working.
Medical	Severe pain	This must always be discussed with the doctor first.
Medical	Thrombosis	Mobile blood clots, usually within the veins deep within the leg. Improved blood circulation can cause clots to break up and move faster. Treatment could also interfere with the uptake of any medications.

Skin irritation

The skin will react very quickly, often going red, becoming itchy and possibly inflamed. Essential oils are very concentrated, which is why the potential for irritating the skin exists. The oils that are most likely to cause an irritation if they are present in a blend in large amounts include cinnamon, clove, fennel, oregano, parsley seed and thyme.

Sensitisation

As with a skin irritation, the sensitisation reaction involves rashes, blotchiness, possibly slight blistering and the development of an allergic-style reaction (so the skin will react more violently if the essential oil in question is used again). Most of the essential oils that are known to be sensitisers are not commercially available; however there are a few essential oils that are considered to offer a slight risk of sensitisation (and might therefore be best avoided if you know that you have very sensitive skin). These include lemongrass, may chang, melissa, myrrh and ylang ylang.

Idiosyncratic reaction

This is an allergic-style reaction to an essential oil or a carrier oil that is generally not regarded as an allergen. When something like this happens, the only thing you can do is remove the product from the person's skin immediately, and always patch test anything new when treating them in the future. Sometimes the reaction can be surprising – for example, I have seen one person react in this way to lavender oil.

casestudy: What to do if someone has hypersensitive skin

Apart from having an immaculate complexion, Denise has a wide range of sensitivities to foods and to various skin products. She came along to a class on natural facials which involved using some of the facial masks outlined on pages 68–71. Unfortunately, there were a couple to which she reacted badly: the banana mask (she is allergic to bananas anyway and commented afterwards that she really should have known better than to cover her face in banana) and the honey and coconut mask (this was more surprising). Her skin reacted to the products by quickly becoming hot and then itchy. In both instances, it was necessary to wash off the offending products immediately with plain cool water and pat the skin dry afterwards. Lavender, German chamomile or yarrow essential oils can remove the pain, itchiness and inflammation from a skin reaction, although in Denise's case we had access to some plain aloe vera gel, which was more appropriate, given the immediacy of her response. On both occasions, the inflammation cleared completely within five minutes.

The rest of the class, meanwhile, had no problems with the masks in question, despite the fact that other participants also had sensitive skin. Denise found that the best mask for her was the plain avocado mask (see page 71).

FAQs – About contraindications

I'm concerned about using aromatherapy at all for my friend, who is pregnant, but she is suffering from very bad nausea – are there any oils that could help her?

You can help her by giving her a tissue with a couple of drops of essential oil on it for her to sniff. Use very few drops, as her sense of smell is very strong right now. Good essential oils to try in order to combat nausea include lemon, grapefruit, geranium, rosewood, patchouli, ginger, black pepper or peppermint. Try one drop each of lemon and rosewood.

I've just found out that I'm pregnant, and I've been using essential oils at full strength in blends designed to enhance my fertility! Will this harm my baby?

No, it won't. Even the full strength blends are generally okay as the essential oils you will have used to enhance your fertility are among the safest we use. However, once you are pregnant, your skin becomes more sensitive and more porous. Your sense of smell will be a lot stronger too. You may find that the essential oils that you previously enjoyed are now much too strong and may even worsen any nausea you are experiencing! Once you know you are pregnant, and *if* you feel strongly that you wish to continue using aromatherapy during your first trimester, you must reduce the amount of essential oils down to one per cent in solution. If you have a history of unstable pregnancies (or, if this is your first pregnancy and/or there is a family history of unstable pregnancies) then I strongly recommend that you avoid putting essential oils on your skin until you are safely through your first trimester.

How do you know that 2 per cent in 20 mls is eight drops of essential oil? Surely not all droppers are the same size? (And did someone really research this?)

Actually, yes, a few years ago someone did take the trouble to analyse the size and shape of all the droppers currently available and to check that we really do provide the essential oils at the correct dilution. You are right, there are some vagaries in the measuring system, but it has stood the test as a reasonable method of use. You really do have to take the trouble of carefully counting the drops of essential oil you add to a blend. If you accidentally add more than you intended to, add more carrier oil accordingly (and measure that out correctly, too). As to the maths, this works on the basis that there are 20 drops in 1 ml of any essential oil. So a 100 per cent solution in 20 ml would be $20 \times 20 = 400$ drops. A 2 per cent solution in 20 ml of carrier oil $= 2/100 \times 400 = 8$ drops.

Does photosensitisation mean that if I put bergamot oil on my skin and then go on the sunbed I'll get a deeper, more long lasting tan?

No it doesn't; you will burn, perhaps badly. If you love the smell of bergamot, you can reduce the number of drops of the essential oil in your blend, so that it is present in your blend at less than one per cent (which means you have less than four drops of bergamot in your blend at 20 ml of carrier oil), but I would steer clear of using the sunbed after applying your blend anyway, especially if you have sensitive skin.

aromatherapy techniques

Most of us associate aromatherapy with massage. Massage is one of the most effective ways of getting the essential oils into the body and for the person to enjoy the therapeutic benefits of both the essential oils and of the massage. In this section, you will find a basic aromatherapy massage sequence, as well as instructions for blending essential oils in massage oil.

However, aromatherapy doesn't stop there; we'll also be looking at some other aromatherapy techniques that you can use to improve your health and even clean your home.

creating an aromatherapy blend

The beauty of aromatherapy lies in the creation of blends. Professional aromatherapists are required to learn exhaustive amounts of information about the benefits and indications of each essential oil when they undergo their training. They are then faced with the same issues as the lay person: Which essential oil to choose from the large array of appropriate ones? Which oils to put together to create a synergistic blend, whether the combination has a more powerful and profound effect on the person being treated than the individual essential oils would have separately?

Choosing the 'right' essential oils

The decision a professional therapist makes depends on experience: what they know has worked in the past for similar conditions, or where other clients have provided similar details in consultations. They also take into account specific guidelines set down in their training. They may also take an intuitive leap. Over the years I have seen therapists choose effective blends using the following techniques:

- Choosing from a list of essential oils appropriate for each of the conditions the client is presenting. The final blend will be made up of essential oils that were common across the conditions.

- Establishing the number of drops to be used of each of the chosen essential oils, based on either the strength of its chemical constituents or by using a 'blending factor', which indicates the relative strength of its fragrance.

- Short-listing appropriate essential oils, then using muscle-testing techniques borrowed from applied kinesiology to select the best essential oils for the client on the day.

- Short-listing appropriate essential oils, then using a pendulum to make the final decision as to which is best for the client.

- Short-listing appropriate essential oils, then making the final decision based on the use of the five element theory (an aspect of Traditional Chinese Medicine (TCM) that is also central to an understanding of feng shui) and an understanding of any energetic imbalances (in the five elements) the client is presenting.

- Short-listing appropriate essential oils, then making a decision based on the principals of Ayurvedic medicine and the understanding of the dosha appropriate to the client.

- Short-listing appropriate essential oils, then blending using the concepts of perfumery – choosing a top, middle and base note to create a rounded and fragrant blend.

Learning to smell essential oils

The blends suggested throughout this book are ones that have been tried and tested on the basis of the appropriateness of the oils for the conditions concerned. However, as you get to know each of the essential oils you will be introduced to, you might like to try doing a smell test and thinking about the essential oils in terms of their top, middle and base notes. Here's how that works.

Conducting a smell test on an essential oil:

1 Place a drop of the essential oil on a cotton bud, tissue or a smelling strip.

2 Smell it immediately (just waft it back and forth under your nose, don't sniff heavily) for the first 30 seconds after the essential oil is exposed to the air. Write down any observations you have of the essential oil at this time. Think about any sensations you feel in your body (where might the essential oil affect you?) as well as any emotional response you have to the oil. This represents the essential oil's top note.

3 Leave the essential oil for a couple of minutes then go back and smell it again. Think about how it has changed over time. Do you feel any different about it? Do you like the smell more, or less? This represents the essential oil's middle note.

4 Smell the essential oil after eight minutes and note any additional changes. This is the essential oil's base note.

When perfumers design a new fragrance, they use essential oils to develop the scent. They take into account not only the individual essential oil's top, middle and base notes as they change over time, but also class an essential oil as a top, middle or base note depending on its fragrance and its volatility (how quickly it evaporates and, effectively, disappears).

In doing the smell test, you have experienced a little of what it is like to consider how volatile an essential oil is. When you smelled the top note, you smelled the essential oil with all of its chemical constituents present. Very quickly, some of these constituents will evaporate (the top notes), so that what you smell next is an indication of some of the less volatile constituents (the middle notes) and finally, the least volatile and most longlasting constituents (the bottom notes).

Question

Consider all of the essential oils you have experimented with. Which would you class as:

- top notes (disappear quickly, they tend to be very uplifting and euphoric)?

- middle notes (last longer, often are quite balancing)?

base notes (last the longest, often smell quite earthy or do not change much over time, may be considered grounding or warming)?

When you do a smell test, describing the essential oil as if it is a wine can also be very effective at helping you to remember the smell and to create a blend that works for you. The first column of the table below lists some of the terms used in the wine industry to describe the characteristics of wine. The second column applies the term to essential oils.

Term used to describe wine	Applied to essential oil
Camphoraceous	Smells medicinal, sometimes painfully so (your nose might itch if you sniff hard)
Floral	Smells of flowers
Fruity	Smells of fruits (usually associated with citrus essential oils, but some of the other essential oils will have fruity notes, possibly as top or middle notes when you do the smell test)
Green	Smells like cut grass, like a garden in the shade
Herbaceous	Smells like garden herbs, particularly when the sun is shining on the foliage
Spicy	Gives a sensation like the taste of spices in food
Woody	Smells like wood
Earthy	Smells like leaf mould or a damp forest

When you start to experiment with essential oils, it is a good idea not to use more than three or four essential oils in a blend until you begin to feel more confident about the blends that you create. Another very useful technique is to create your blend one step at a time:

- Start by measuring out your carrier product (for example, oil, moisturiser, shampoo) and selecting the bottles of essential oil you intend to use.

- Add one drop of essential oil, mixing it thoroughly into the carrier and smelling it before you move on to add a drop from your second essential oil.

- Mix thoroughly after each addition and use your sense of smell to adjust the number of drops of each essential oil until you reach a fragrance and potency that is appropriate to your needs. It is interesting to note that the majority of students who try this end up with a blend containing less than the maximum number of allowable drops.

The essential oils

The following essential oils are among the most readily available and most popular ones to start experimenting with. For the most part, they are relatively inexpensive, the exceptions being rose, neroli and sandalwood. However, brief details of these are included as they smell so beautiful that it is likely that you will want to buy them soon, if not immediately.

A price rating is given from 1 to 5, with 5 being the most expensive.

Name: Benzoin
Botanical name: *Styrax benzoin*
Maximum number of drops: 2 in 20 ml of carrier oil
Useful for: cracked skin, chest infections, catarrh, bronchitis, psoriasis, sinusitis, impetigo, insomnia, anxiety, panic attacks
Cautions/contraindications: none
Blends well with: frankincense, sandalwood, cedarwood, orange, grapefruit, neroli, rose, vetiver, cypress, myrrh, lemon, ylang ylang, Roman chamomile, palmarosa
Price rating: 3

Name: Bergamot
Botanical name: *Citrus bergamia*
Maximum number of drops: 4 in 20 ml of carrier oil

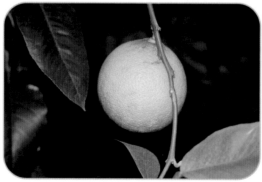

Bergamot

Useful for: acne vulgaris, boils, eczema, dermatitis, psoriasis, abdominal bloating, nausea, thrush, gingivitis, anxiety, depression, lethargy (particularly valuable for stress-related sensitive skin)
Cautions/contraindications: phototoxic – do not use immediately before going on a sunbed or outside into bright sunlight without covering up. Reduce the number of drops of bergamot in a blend when it is sunny and cover up after applying the oil to your skin
Blends well with: cedarwood, lavender, marjoram, clary sage, coriander, frankincense, ginger, grapefruit, lemon, neroli, nutmeg, orange, patchouli, peppermint, pine, petitgrain, sandalwood, vetiver
Price rating: 2

Name: Cedarwood
Botanical name: *Cedrus atlantic, Cedrus deodar, Juniperus virginiana*

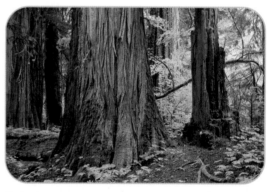

Cedar tree

Three varieties are commonly available: cedarwood Atlas (*Cedrus atlantica*), Himalayan cedarwood (*Cedrus deodar*) and Virginian cedarwood (*Juniperus virginiana*). All are very useful for skin conditions, with the first two having a slightly more floral odour, whilst the latter smells far more antiseptic. Conditions and blending recommendations below assume that you have chosen either Atlas or Himalayan cedarwood.

Maximum number of drops: 2 in 20 ml of carrier oil

Useful for: asthma, eczema, psoriasis, acne, dry skin, infected skin, ingrown hairs, dandruff

Cautions/contraindications: none

Blends well with: lavender, sandalwood, Roman chamomile, German chamomile, yarrow, lemon, frankincense, cypress, neroli, rose, jasmine, ylang ylang, vetiver, bergamot, patchouli, palmarosa, lemongrass, pine, niaouli, coriander

Price rating: 3

Name: Cypress
Botanical name: *Cupressus sempervirens*

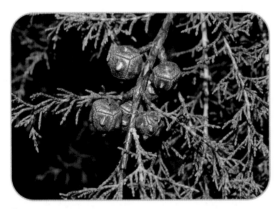

Cypress tree

Maximum number of drops: 2 in 20 ml of carrier oil

Useful for: excessive sweating, thread veins, red veins, varicose veins, haemorrhoids, cellulite, oedema

Cautions/contraindications: none

Blends well with: lemon, rosemary, grapefruit, juniper, orange, neroli, bergamot, palmarosa, lavender, geranium

Price rating: 3

Name: Frankincense
Botanical name: *Boswellia carterii*

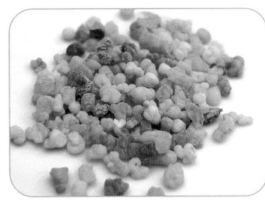

Frankincense resin

Maximum number of drops: 3 in 20 ml of carrier oil

Useful for: dry, mature, wrinkled skin, eczema, psoriasis, coughs, colds, influenza, as well as muscular aches and pains

Cautions/contraindications: none

Blends well with: cedarwood, sandalwood, benzoin, myrrh, black pepper, bergamot, lemon, orange, neroli, rose, lavender, grapefruit, Roman chamomile, cypress

Price rating: 4

Name: Geranium
Botanical name: *Pelargonium graveolens*. There are two varieties – geranium and rose geranium. The latter is a very common ingredient of cosmetic products and has also been used to adulterate rose otto as the fragrance of geranium has some similarities to the more expensive rose.

Maximum number of drops: 3 in 20 ml of carrier oil

Useful for: hormonally-sensitive skin (skin that is prone to blemishes as a result of changes in the menstural cycle or in testosterone levels), oedema, lymphatic congestion, ringworm, psoriasis, athlete's foot, anxiety, depression, itchy or inflamed skin, irregular or painful menstruation, as a hormonal regulator at menopause, during pregnancy, for endometriosis, fibroids, sexual disinterest, nervous exhaustion, digestive difficulties including IBS, constipation

Cautions/contraindications: none

Blends well with: cedarwood, Roman chamomile, clary sage, coriander, fennel, frankincense, ginger, grapefruit, lemon, neroli, nutmeg, orange, patchouli, peppermint, petitgrain, sandalwood, vetiver

Price rating: 2

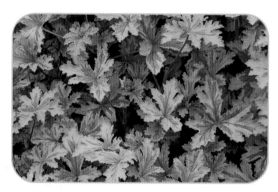

Geranium

Name: Juniper

Botanical name: *Juniperus officinalis*

Maximum number of drops: 2 in 20 ml of carrier oil

Useful for: oedema, infected acne, blemishes, cellulite, any form of detoxification

Cautions/contraindications: strong diuretic – be careful if the person is already using diuretics or has a history of kidney disorders

Blends well with: orange, grapefruit, cedarwood, rosemary, cypress, lavender,

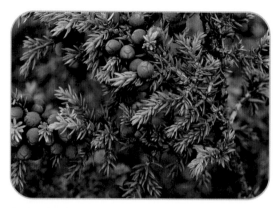

Juniper berries

marjoram, fennel, lemongrass, lemon, mandarin, tangerine, vetiver, rose

Price rating: 3

Name: Lavender

Botanical name: *Lavandula angustifolia.* Other varieties of lavender exist and include those with the common names of spike lavender, lavandin, lavender cotton. Make sure you get the *angustifolia* variety as this is the safest one to use and is not contraindicated for any condition.

Maximum number of drops: 4 in 20 ml of carrier oil

Useful for: everything! Use lavender first for insomnia, cuts, eczema, asthma, psoriasis, burns, insect bites and stings, infected skin conditions, muscular aches and pains, pain in

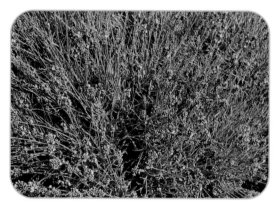

Lavender

the TMJ (temporalmandibular joint), high blood pressure, headaches, migraines, nausea, thrush and cystitis, athlete's foot.

Cautions/contraindications: none

Blends well with: cedarwood, bergamot, sandalwood, rose, rosemary, neroli, orange, lemon, vetiver, patchouli, lemongrass, cypress, myrrh, marjoram, peppermint, yarrow, Roman chamomile, German chamomile, tangerine, mandarin, grapefruit

Price rating: 1

Name: Lemon
Botanical name: *Citrus limonum*

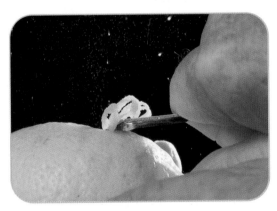

Lemon

Maximum number of drops: 4 in 20 ml of carrier oil

Useful for: warts, veruccas, fungal infections, viral infections, ME, post-viral fatigue, lack of concentration, SAD (seasonal affective disorder), broken capillaries, thread veins, allergic reactions, insect bites and stings, rashes, cellulite, constipation, headaches, lethargy

Cautions/contraindications: mildly phototoxic

Blends well with: cedarwood, Roman chamomile, clary sage, coriander, fennel, frankincense, ginger, grapefruit, lemon, neroli, nutmeg, orange, patchouli, peppermint, petitgrain, sandalwood, vetiver

Price rating: 1

Name: Mandarin
Botanical name: *Citrus reticulata*

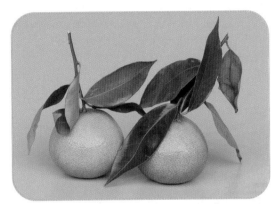

Mandarin

Maximum number of drops: 4 in 20 ml of carrier oil

Useful for: digestive upsets (including flatulence, constipation, colic), insomnia, anxiety, nightmares, cellulite (mildly effective), lymphatic congestion

Cautions/contraindications: very safe – recommended for use with babies and during pregnancy

Blends well with: lavender, neroli, petitgrain, vetiver, juniper, orange, lemon, marjoram, sandalwood, rosewood, ginger, lemongrass

Price rating: 2

Name: Myrrh
Botanical name: *Comiphora myrrha*
Maximum number of drops: 2 in 20 ml of carrier oil

Useful for: coughs with mucous, rhinitis, sinusitis, facial rejuvenation (reduces wrinkles), arthritis, amenorrhoea, insomnia, damaged skin, athlete's foot, haemorrhoids
Cautions/contraindications: none
Blends well with: frankincense, cedarwood, sandalwood, marjoram, bergamot, lavender, orange, palmarosa, vetiver, rose, neroli, jasmine
Price rating: 3

Name: Neroli
Botanical name: *Citrus aurantium*
Maximum number of drops: 3 in 20 ml of carrier oil

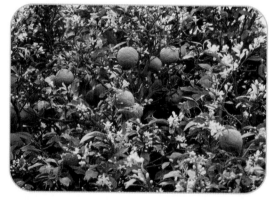

Neroli

Useful for: shock, very sensitive skin, stress-related sensitive skin, heart conditions, nervous diarrhoea, stress-related digestive difficulties, preventing or reducing signs of stretch marks, reducing wrinkling in dry, dehydrated or mature skin
Cautions/contraindications: none
Blends well with: cedarwood, Roman chamomile, clary sage, coriander, Damiana, fennel, frankincense, ginger, grapefruit, lemon, neroli, nutmeg, orange, patchouli, peppermint, petitgrain, sandalwood, vetiver
Price rating: 5

Name: Orange
Botanical name: *Citrus aurantium var. sinensis* – different varieties available including mandarin (*Citrus reticulata*), and Shamouti orange (smells like Jaffa orange). All carry out roughly the same functions as listed below and are safe to use in the same dosage, but smell slightly different – choose the one you like the best.

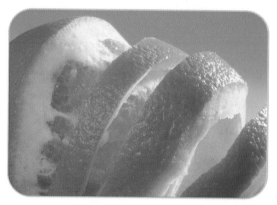

Orange

Maximum number of drops: 2 in 20 ml of carrier oil
Useful for: insomnia, indigestion, nightmares, anxiety, acne, dermatitis, thread veins, reduces fluid retention. Safe to use on infants and small children in small amounts
Cautions/contraindications: Mildly phototoxic
Blends well with: cedarwood, sandalwood, frankincense, petitgrain, fennel, vetiver, neroli, jasmine, benzoin, ginger
Price rating: 1

Name: Palmarosa
Botanical name: *Cymbopogon martini*
Maximum number of drops: 2 in 20 mls
Useful for: acne, dermatitis, infected skin, nervousness, insecurity, to cool and calm anger, constipation, sluggish digestion, as an insect repellent, to reduce fevers

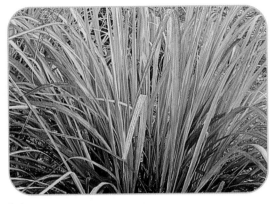

Palmarosa

good for inflamed conditions and for chronic insomnia but smells quite medicinal.

Maximum number of drops: 2 in 20 ml of carrier oil

Useful for: asthma, eczema, psoriasis, insomnia, anxiety, neuralgia, painful periods, toothache, burns, IBS

Cautions/contraindications: none

Blends well with: clary sage, black pepper, sandalwood, lavender, marjoram, rosemary, thyme, palmarosa, vetiver, rose, bergamot, orange, grapefruit, cedarwood

Price rating: 4

Blends well with: patchouli, rosewood, rose, geranium, lemon, orange, petitgrain, ginger, frankincense, neroli, Roman chamomile, lemongrass, melissa, vetiver, black pepper

Price rating: 2–3

Name: Rose otto

Botanical name: *Rosa damascaena, Rosa centifolia*

Maximum number of drops: 2 in 20 ml of carrier oil

Name: Roman chamomile

Botanical name: *Anthemis nobilis.* Several different varieties of chamomile are available,

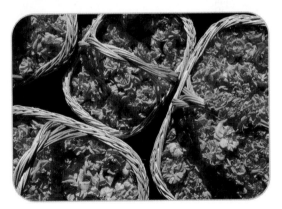

Rose otto

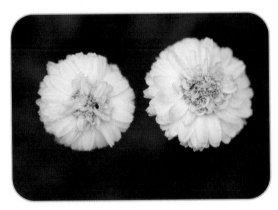

Roman chamomile

including Chamomile maroc (*Ormenis multicaulis*) and German (or blue) chamomile (*Chamomila matricaria*). Roman chamomile has a sweeter and gentler fragrance, which is more appropriate for use on the face and with children. German chamomile is extremely

Useful for: cold sores, itchy or inflamed skin, irregular or painful menstruation, as a hormonal regulator at menopause, in the last trimester of pregnancy (to prepare for labour), for endometriosis, fibroids, cirrhosis, addiction, stress-related immune conditions, anger, jealousy, sexual disinterest, nervous exhaustion

Cautions/contraindications: mild emmenagogue. Avoid in first trimester of pregnancy if the person has a history of miscarriages.

Blends well with: cedarwood, Roman chamomile, clary sage, coriander, fennel, frankincense, ginger, grapefruit, lemon, neroli, nutmeg, orange, patchouli, peppermint, petitgrain, sandalwood, vetiver
Price rating: 5

Name: Rosemary
Botanical name: *Rosmarinus officinalis*
Maximum number of drops: 2 in 20 ml of carrier oil

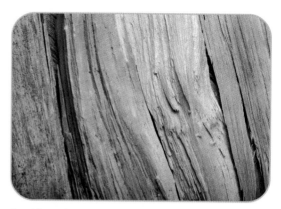
Sandalwood

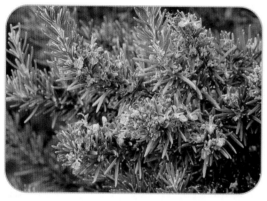
Rosemary

Useful for: acne or dry skin – balances hormonally-sensitive skin, eczema, psoriasis, cystitis, coughs with mucous, sore throats, chronic bronchitis, cold sores, tonsillitis, earaches, sinusitis, to support asthma. Mildly sedating.
Cautions/contraindications: none
Blends well with: cedarwood, Roman chamomile, coriander, frankincense, ginger, grapefruit, lemon, neroli, orange, patchouli, petitgrain, vetiver, lavender, marjoram, benzoin, tea tree, jasmine
Price rating: 3–5, depending on variety

Useful for: low blood pressure, poor circulation, muscular aches and pains, acne vulgaris, excessively oily skin, sinusitis, rhinitis, coughs, colds, bronchitis, mental fatigue
Cautions/contraindications: avoid where someone has epilepsy, high blood pressure, or is pregnant. Stimulant, so avoid before sleep.
Blends well with: orange, lemon, marjoram, lavender, grapefruit, frankincense, myrrh, palmarosa, lemongrass, black pepper
Price rating: 2

Name: Tea tree
Botanical name: *Melaleuca alternifolia*
Maximum number of drops: 3 in 20 ml of carrier oil

Name: Sandalwood
Botanical name: *Santalum album*, from Mysore in India, or *Santalum spicatum* – Australian sandalwood (now more commonly available).
Maximum number of drops: 2 in 20 ml of carrier oil

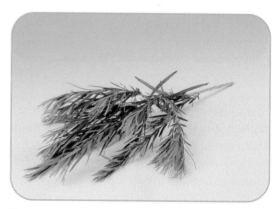
Tea tree

Useful for: athlete's foot, insect bites and stings, cuts, infected eczema, infected acne, acne vulgaris, cold sores, nailbed infections, thrush, ringworm, impetigo.

Cautions/contraindications: none – but is not always recommended if you are having homeopathic treatment

Blends well with: peppermint, bergamot, eucalyptus, lavender, rosemary, lemon, grapefruit, marjoram

Price rating: 1

Name: Vetiver

Botanical name: *Vetiveria zizanoides*

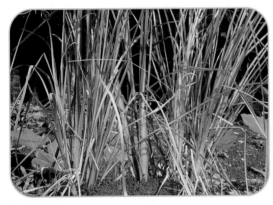
Vetiver

Maximum number of drops: 2 in 20 ml of carrier oil

Useful for: lymphatic congestion, detoxification, pain in TMJ or muscular aches and pains, as an ingredient in any products designed for men,

Cautions/contraindications: none

Blends well with: neroli, rose, jasmine, geranium, nutmeg, orange, lavender, Roman chamomile, sandalwood, cedarwood, yarrow, ylang ylang, bergamot, grapefruit, lemon, palmarosa

Price rating: 3

Name: Ylang ylang

Botanical name: *Cananga odorata*

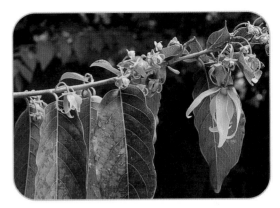
Ylang ylang

Maximum number of drops: 2 in 20 ml of carrier oil

Useful for: anxiety, depression, sexual disinterest, to help control epileptic seizures, heart palpitations, anger, shock, rage, frustration, stress, high blood pressure, thread veins, chapped or dry skin

Cautions/contraindications: none – but note that it is very effective at lowering blood pressure, so do not use on someone who has low blood pressure, unless you are mixing it with an oil that will help to maintain or raise blood pressure

Blends well with: cedarwood, Roman chamomile, clary sage, coriander, fennel, frankincense, ginger, grapefruit, lemon, neroli, orange, patchouli, petitgrain, sandalwood, vetiver

Price rating: 1

Aromatherapy and feng shui

Feng shui is the ancient Chinese discipline of placement. It is based on the belief that the arrangement of your home, your desk, your workplace and your environment can influence every aspect of your life. Feng shui can be used to enhance your career, your relationships, your finances and your health and much more.

A concept which is central to feng shui is five element theory. This suggests that all the life energy surrounding us and governing our lives (and personal health) works in a cycle that we can compare to the seasons:

- Fire – the height of summer, exciting, zesty, dynamic, uplifting

- Earth – the abundance of harvest, earthiness, substance and feelings of abundance and satisfaction

- Metal – the depth of winter, cool, cold, crisp: things are dormant and waiting for spring

- Water – early spring, when the rains are abundant, watery, cool, clear (April showers)

- Wood – when trees and plants start to grow quickly, things are warming up, clear spring days (May flowers).

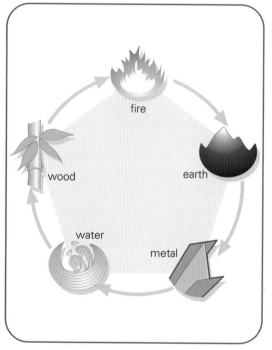

The five elements in the productive cycle

Try this

Try putting the essential oils you have smelled into one of these five element categories, based on how they make you feel. Now imagine how you could use this to create a blend for the vaporiser. What would you use if the room felt hot and stuffy and needed cooling down? What about in the middle of winter when everyone around you is complaining about the cold?

You may also want to compare your findings with those outlined by Gabriel Mojay in his book *Aromatherapy for Healing the Spirit*, (2005) which links aromatherapy with Traditional Chinese Medicine (TCM also relies on the five element theory).

casestudy: Festive fear

Marianne dreaded the Christmas period. She has a large extended family to buy gifts for and provides lunch for them all on Christmas day. This year, there was more potential than usual for arguments, due to family disagreement. Marianne was also on a tight budget. She decided to make everyone aromatherapy products to suit their personal interests (and also to promote a calm atmosphere). She came up with the following blends, which she added to bubble bath, moisturiser or shower gel.

For the boys, she put together a blend designed to lower testosterone and aggression levels:

- marjoram 2 drops
- benzoin 3 drops
- cedarwood 2 drops
- bergamot 1 drop

in 20 ml of carrier product.

For the girls, she decided to prepare a blend designed to promote calm:

- benzoin 2 drops
- geranium 3 drops
- cypress 3 drops

in 20 ml of carrier product.

Marianne also created a blend to use in the vaporiser to fragrance the house before everyone arrived, which she kept going throughout the festivities. She reported that everyone liked her blend so much, she made up bottles of it for her guests to take home, too!

For the vaporiser:

- benzoin 4
- pine 2
- nutmeg 1
- orange 3.

The result was a success – everyone was pleased with their aromatherapy gifts, there was far less arguing than usual and Marianne was able to watch her favourite films in peace.

FAQs — About creating a blend

I don't know what I'm doing wrong, but my blends always seem to smell strange. What can I do to make them more pleasant?

Try working out which element of your current blends smells strange. Is it an odd combination? Have you been using the same essential oil for a long period of time, putting it in everything you make? If that's the case, your body may be rebelling and asking for a change. If the blend smells fine before it is put on the skin, but odd when it is on, it could be down to food just eaten by the person wearing the blend. Strong flavours, including garlic and some spices, are excreted in the sweat and when they blend with the essential oils on the skin, result in an unpleasant smell.

What am I doing wrong? My blends tend to smell great at first, but the fragrance doesn't last.

There are a couple of possibilities. You may be using a poor quality essential oil. It may be close to the end of its shelf life, or it may have been stored in a warm environment or under lights. It could be that it is the result of a poor harvest. Also, it is possible that you have put mostly 'top notes' in your blend, with essential oils that are more likely to evaporate faster. If this is likely, try changing the oils you are using to always include those in which the fragrance lasts a little longer (the woods and resins, for example). The citrus oils and florals such as neroli appear to be the most volatile, evaporating very quickly.

bases for
blending

Essential oils surround us in our daily lives. A trip around the average supermarket will show you that they are added to many products: they flavour foods; form the basis of perfumes; and are found in our deodorants, lip balms, bathing products, candles, dish-washing liquids, household cleaning products and air fresheners.

Designing your own aromatherapy products is one of the most enjoyable aspects of working with aromatherapy. Carrier oils, unperfumed base products and containers are easily available (see the stockists listed at the end of this book). The only thing that could hold you back is a lack of imagination.

Making your own products

Here are just some of the things you can easily create:

- body massage oil
- facial oil
- hair oil
- facial products
- perfumes
- shower gel
- bubble bath
- bath oils
- compresses

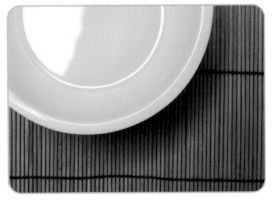

Carrier oil

41

🔖 exfoliants

🔖 room vaporisers

🔖 inhalations

🔖 for laundry.

Body massage oil

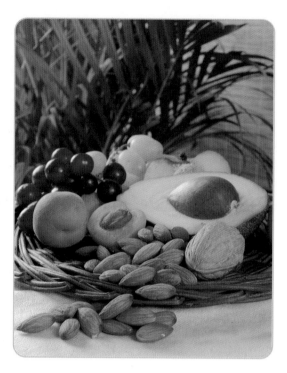

Oil is probably the most common medium in which to blend essential oils and is required if you are going to carry out an aromatherapy massage. These oils are referred to as carrier oils, base oils or, sometimes, fixed oils. The choice of massage oil can also help to improve the health of the individual and particularly their skin. The following table gives you some details about the most common carrier oils available.

A price rating is given, from 1 to 5, with 5 being the most expensive.

Carrier oils

Carrier oil	Features	Price rating
Jojoba	Antibacterial, chemically similar to sebum. Sebum will dissolve in jojoba. Use on all skin types, especially sensitive, dry, dehydrated, or where eczema, acne or psoriasis exist. Can also be used to remove make up. Very useful for the scalp when treating dandruff or cradle cap.	4
Avocado	Anti-inflammatory, some sunscreen properties, use for eczema and for dehydrated, mature and environmentally sensitive skin types. Use unrefined avocado oil by preference (it has a distinctive greenish colour).	4
Hazelnut	Mildly astringent, stimulates circulation. Use for oily, acne vulgaris, or hormonally and stress-related sensitive skin. Avoid in cases of acne rosacea.	3
Macadamia nut	As for jojoba, chemically similar to sebum. Good for dry and mature skin.	4
Peach kernel	Useful for normal, dry, dehydrated and sensitive skins, pleasant fragrance, slightly richer than sweet almond but has similar properties.	2

Carrier oil	Features	Price rating
Calendula	Anti-inflammatory, reduces scar tissue, use for dehydrated, damaged or irritated skin, including chapped skin and cracked heels. Helps skin to heal quickly and efficiently. Very useful at helping to prevent and to repair stretch marks, it also has a mild toning effect on the veins, so it is very useful as a carrier oil when dealing with thread veins, varicose veins and haemorrhoids, or where mild inflammation exists.	3
Sweet almond	Use for chapped, inflamed or irritated skin and where there is eczema or dermatitis. Useful for normal or dry skin types.	2
Evening primrose	Use for skin that is dry, oily or affected by acne, for hormonally-sensitive skin. Helps to rebalance sebum secretions, mildly anti-inflammatory (try adding it to blends for arthritis and any inflamed skin conditions). Use for eczema, psoriasis or poor hair or nail conditions. A very useful carrier oil to include if the person you are treating is experiencing hormone-related problems such as PMT or menopausal symptoms. Generally sold in capsule form. Simply pierce capsule and add to another carrier oil.	5
Coconut	Relieves dry and itching skin. Use for dry, cracked, mature or environmentally sensitive skin. Monoi de Tahiti – a substance found in some baby skincare products – is made of gardenia flowers cold-pressed in coconut oil.	3
Apricot kernel	Calms inflammations, used for eczema, dermatitis, or for dry, mature and sensitive skin	2
Grapeseed	A very useful all-rounder for massage. Hypoallergenic, so a skin reaction to this oil is extremely rare. Usually costs less than most other carrier oils and can be purchased in large amounts in the supermarket (along with sunflower oil).	1
Sunflower	Useful for hormonally-sensitive skin. A good all-rounder. Can easily be found in supermarkets.	1
Argan	Fantastic oil for use on the face, has a well-deserved reputation for preserving and healing skin, reducing the appearance of wrinkles, moisturising and nourishing the skin. (Difficult to find in its natural state – you need to go to a wholesalers for it – see resources list at the end of this book.)	5
Wheatgerm	High in nutrients, moisturising, cytophylactic. Good for dry or mature skin. Avoid where there is a possibility of wheat intolerances or where skin is environmentally sensitive. Wheatgerm can help to increase the shelf-life of a blend if it is at 25% of the solution (so 20 ml of carrier oil could include 5 ml of wheatgerm), but on its own it tends to go rancid very quickly. Store it in the fridge.	4

Facial oil

Blends specifically for the face tend to involve using some of the richer, more expensive carrier oils such as argan, evening primrose, avocado and jojoba. As a rule, it is best to stick to a total of 2 per cent essential oils over the entire body, so if you are blending separately to treat the face (but are treating the body at the same time), use one drop of essential oil in 5 ml of carrier oil for the face, and use the other seven drops of essential oil in 15–20 ml carrier oil for the body. If you are planning to treat the face only, you could blend at the same concentration as you would use for the body. However, I find it is preferable to lower the dosage.

For wrinkles:

- frankincense 1 drop
- sandalwood 1 drop
- rose 2 drops

in 20 ml of carrier oil.

For dehydrated skin:

- palmarosa 2 drops
- vetiver 1 drop
- rose 1 drop

in 20 ml of jojoba/avocado or argan oil.

For oily skin:

- lemon 2 drops
- cypress 1 drop
- geranium 1 drop

in 20 ml of carrier oil.

For Acne vulgaris:

- rose 1 drop
- lemon 2 drops
- juniper 1 drop

in 20 ml of carrier oil.

Hair oil

If your hair has been ravaged by chemicals, the weather, or drying equipment, a hair oil treatment is an incredibly relaxing and effective (if messy) way to return it to its former glory. For these treatments, use the same carrier oils that you would use for body massage, but halve the number of drops of essential oil in the blend (use a maximum of 4 drops in 20 ml of carrier oil for a healthy adult). This is because the skin of the scalp is more porous than the skin elsewhere, so essential oils will penetrate faster. For the best effects, apply the hair oil (warming it is optional) to dry hair, wrap the hair in a plastic shower cap (or in cling film) then a towel (to keep it warm). Leave for at least an hour, before applying shampoo (Note: do *not* add

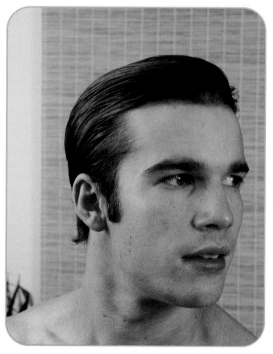

Protecting the hair

water before you add the shampoo). Use enough shampoo to build up a light lather, then add water to clean all the oil out of your hair. Shampoo and condition as normal. Camellia is widely used as the carrier oil for this treatment in Japan. In India, coconut oil is a favourite, especially if jasmine has been cold-pressed in it. Carrier oils that are particularly beneficial for split ends include calendula, evening primrose and apricot kernel.

For dandruff:

- cypress 2 drops
- lavender 1 drop
- cedarwood 1 drop

in 20 ml of carrier oil.

For hair loss:

- rosemary 1 drop
- cedarwood 2 drops
- lemon 1 drop

in 20 ml carrier oil.

For blonde hair:

- lemon 2 drops
- Roman chamomile 2 drops

in 20 ml carrier oil.

These are the essential oils traditionally used to bring additional highlights to blonde hair. There is no guarantee that you will see spectacular results from using this hair oil,

but it does seem to help remove any residue that might dull the hair.

As part of a luxury home spa experience:

- sandalwood 2 drops
- jasmine 1 drop
- melissa (or lemon if you prefer) 1 drop

in 20 ml of carrier oil.

Shampoos and conditioners

As with the hair oil treatment, it is advisable to keep the essential oils used in shampoos and conditioners down to 4 drops in 20 mls.

Facial products

When you are creating a range of facial products, it is important to consider how they will be used. If the user will be using only one aromatherapy product on their face, then you can blend up to 2 per cent (so a moisturiser might contain eight drops of essential oil in 20 ml of moisturising base). However, I prefer to use a maximum of 4–5 drops.

If, however, the person will be using a cleanser, toner *and* moisturiser containing aromatherapy oils, it is advisable to ensure that you blend at significantly lower doses. If you are making all three products, ensure that the eight drops of essential oil are spread among the three, with the majority of the essential oils appearing in the product that will be on their skin for the longest time. For example:

	At 2 per cent	At 1 per cent
Cleanser	2 drops	1 drop
Toner	1 drop	0 drops
Moisturiser	5 drops	3 drops

Please note that this represents a significantly lower percentage of essential oils in the products than you would find in any commercially available product. However, your safety and the safety of the person you are treating must be considered. Commercially available products are all extensively tested.

Cleanser

A wide range of different types and styles of cleansing products is available. For your purposes, a fragrance-free, cream-based cleanser is the most useful for blending. For sole use (when you are producing only the cleanser) a maximum of eight drops in 20 ml is fine. For multiple use, go down to one or two drops in 20 ml.

Essential oils that are particularly useful when cleansing the face include lemon, sandalwood, rosewood, lavender, juniper, tea tree, cedarwood and bergamot.

Toner

Toners are designed to provide a mild astringent effect on the skin, clearing any waste materials and closing pores (or making them appear smaller). You can use hydrolats (flower waters) as toners – rosewater is a particularly lovely one to try. They are especially useful if you have very sensitive or dry skin and tend to react badly to commercially-produced toners, most of which contain alcohol. Occasionally, you may find flower waters with added glycerin. Glycerin can help to soften and moisturise the skin and is particularly useful in toners. Keep essential oils to a minimum in toners, as they do not dissolve easily here. One drop of essential oil in 20 ml of toner is more than sufficient.

- For acne vulgaris – try sandalwood, tea tree, rosemary, lemon, juniper or lavender in toner.
- For acne rosacea – try cedarwood, cypress, geranium, rosewood or palmarosa in toner.

Moisturiser

Cream moisturiser is possibly the most useful product to make if the person you are creating it for is likely to only use one item. The cream helps to form a protective barrier against the elements and, as the product is designed to be applied and then stay on the skin, the effects of the blend on the person will be long lasting. Moisturisers for the face that will be used at night are a particularly useful way of dealing with any sleeping disorders. Work to a maximum of eight drops of essential oil in 20 ml, or less if this is part of a range of products.

Try this:

As well as using a fragrance-free moisturiser to blend in, you can try a very simple method of creating a moisturiser from scratch. Because this blend is made of oil and aloe vera rather than being petroleum-based, it will sink very quickly into the skin.

- 20 ml carrier oil (of your choice – jojoba or avocado are particularly effective)
- 40 ml aloe vera gel.

Whisk thoroughly. For best effects, store in the fridge.

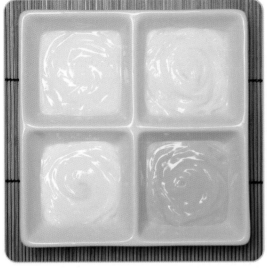

Moisturising gels, made with aloe vera gel. Top left contains coconut oil, top right Argan, bottom left jojoba and bottom right avocado oil.

Citrus for women:

- rosemary 2 drops
- lemon 2 drops
- petitgrain 2 drops
- grapefruit 3 drops
- lavender 3 drops

in 40 ml of perfume base.

Musky for women:

- jasmine 3 drops
- ylang ylang 2 drops
- patchouli 3 drops
- grapefruit 4 drops

in 40 ml of perfume base.

Perfumes

Essential oils partially disperse in alcohol. If you want to make a perfume that you can spray or mist easily onto your body, use water, toner or a hydrolat as a base. To these you can add an unfragranced alcohol (such as vodka or surgical spirit) so that the alcohol is present up to 25 per cent in solution (for example: 15 ml of hydrolat and 5 ml of vodka). If the toner already has alcohol in it, you do not need to add any more. Keep these at a lower dilution than you would use normally and make sure you shake well before each use.

For men:

- vetiver 3 drops
- sandalwood 3 drops
- bergamot 4 drops
- jasmine 2 drops

in 40 ml of perfume base.

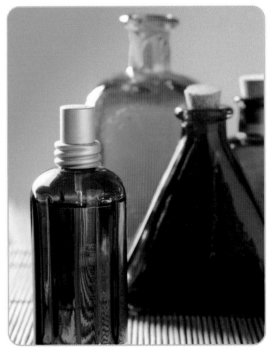

Perfumes

47

Floral innocent:

- neroli 3 drops
- petitgrain 3 drops
- orange 2 drops
- lemon 2 drops
- lavender 2 drops

in 40 ml of perfume base.

Shower gel

Blend up to eight drops in 20 ml of shower gel. Most people tend to prefer zesty, citrus blends as they give a bit of a lift at the start of the day.

To wake up in the morning:

- bergamot 4 drops
- peppermint 2 drops
- lavender 2 drops

in 20 ml of shower gel.

For stress-related eczema:

- lavender 3 drops
- cedarwood 3 drops
- yarrow 2 drops

in 20 ml of shower gel.

Bubble bath

Work up to a maximum of 8 drops in 20 ml of bubble bath base. Blends that are generally preferred are ones that will aid sleep, clear catarrh or ease any muscular aches and pains.

For insomnia:

- marjoram 2 drops
- Roman chamomile 2 drops
- cypress 3 drops
- geranium 1 drops

in 20 ml of bubble bath base.

Muscular aches and pains:

- marjoram 2 drops
- lavender 4 drops
- rosemary 2 drops

in 20 ml of bubble bath base.

Preparation for a night out (or in – this contains three aphrodisiacs)

- neroli 2 drops
- rose 1 drop
- frankincense 2 drops
- black pepper 3 drops

in 20 ml of bubble bath base.

Hangover recovery (heavy on the detoxifying essential oils):

- juniper 3 drops
- lavender 2 drops
- lemon 2 drops
- peppermint 1 drop

in 20 ml of bubble bath base.

Oils for the bath (alone or to share)

If you do not want to add anything but essential oils to your bath, don't add more than six drops. If you tend to have sensitive skin, be very careful about the essential oils that you choose to put in the bath. Avoid all the citrus oils and any essential oils that are noted as making skin prone to sensitisation (for example, lemongrass, melissa, basil, rosemary and eucalyptus can all cause itching). If you are determined to use one or more of these essential oils in the bath, stir them into a cup of whole milk before adding it to the bath. The milk will also soften the skin. Try these.

For anxiety and to cool anger:

- palmarosa 3 drops
- patchouli 2 drops.

For painful periods or menopausal symptoms:

- rose 2 drops
- patchouli 1 drop.

For men (deeply relaxing, but full of aphrodisiacs):

- vetiver 2 drops
- sandalwood 2 drops.

Compresses

Hot and cold compresses can be very useful for everything from muscular aches and pains to muscle strains and sprained knees or ankles. You can enhance the effects of the compress by adding a maximum of two drops of your chosen essential oil to the water in which you are soaking the compress. Useful essential oils for compresses include:

- ginger, peppermint, lavender (for muscle strains/aches and pains)
- lavender, marjoram, chamomile, tea tree (for inflammation).

Exfoliants

You can create very effective yet gentle exfoliants for your hands and feet using sugar or salt. Once you have created the scrubs, they will last for a maximum of six weeks. If you want to make these into beautiful gifts, add plant material (such as lavender flowers, rose petals or similar) to the jar.

For the hands:

- 2 heaped tablespoons sugar
- 30 ml of carrier oil
- 3 drops of essential oil.

For the feet:

- 2 heaped tablespoons salt (use a finely ground salt)
- 30 ml of carrier oil
- 3 drops of essential oil.

For dry feet and cracked heels:

- benzoin 1 drop
- lavender 2 drops.

For age spots:

- lemon 2 drops
- cypress 1 drop.

For warts or veruccas:

- lemon 2 drops
- tea tree 1 drop.

For poor circulation:

- black pepper 2 drops
- rose 1 drop.

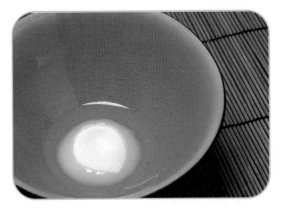

Exfoliant blend

Room vaporisers

Use a maximum of 10 drops in a blend and keep topping up the burner with water. Vaporisers with deep cups to hold the water and essential oils are particularly useful as they will fragrance the room for longer. However, they tend to use tea-light candles to heat the water, so they should not be left burning unattended. Electric burners are safer to use, although they do not have as deep a cup to hold the water.

To clear a room after an argument:

- benzoin 3 drops
- cypress 2 drops
- grapefruit 3 drops.

To provide a meditative atmosphere:

- frankincense 3 drops
- cedarwood 2 drops
- rosewood 3 drops.

To cover cigarette smoke:

- juniper 1 drop
- lemon 4 drops
- lavender 3 drops.

To ease a child's nightmares:

- Roman chamomile 2 drops
- benzoin 4 drops
- orange 2 drops.

Inhalations

Chances are that you have experienced inhalations before – any time you have a chest or head cold and feel the need to clear your sinuses or your lungs. Another use of an inhalation is to steam open the pores on your face prior to a deep cleansing treatment of the skin. Inhalations generally involve using boiling or very hot water in a bowl, to which you would add a maximum of three drops of essential oil (any more will sting your eyes and could leave you feeling nauseous and with a headache). You then place your head over the bowl (and a towel over your head in order to keep the fragrances isolated) and breathe in the fragrant steam for a few minutes.

Popular choices for inhalations are rosemary or eucalyptus, both of which are very effective expectorants, so you can anticipate that coughing will be more productive after using these oils. The following recommendations tend to be more soothing to the chest and nasal passages and are very useful to ensure a clear head as before sleep.

For sinusitis:

- cardamon 2 drops
- lemon 1 drop.

To reduce feelings of 'tight-chestedness' which you know to be associated with a chest cold:

- frankincense 1 drop
- marjoram 1 drop.

To boost the immune system:

- lemongrass 2 drop
- frankincense 1 drop.

To fight chest infections:

- tea tree 1 drop
- cedarwood 3 drops.

To soothe the throat and upper respiratory tract:

- sandalwood 2 drops
- lavender 1 drop.

For laundry

Generations of Britons have used lavender sachets in airing cupboards to fragrance sheets (as well as to keep away moths). You can get similar results by using both essential oils or, if you have access to them, hydrolats, to great effect. (The most readily available hydrolats are rosewater, orange flower water, and lavender water.)

I have found the best way to work with essential oils when doing laundry is to put a drop of essential oil in the jug of water (about 500 ml) to fill the iron. Let the water sit for a few minutes (or up to a day) before you fill the iron. If you can get hold of a hydrolat, that is even more effective. You can dilute the hydrolat down to one part hydrolat to three parts water and still get the unforgettable fragrance on your clothes.

If you are wanting to fragrance clothes that you generally don't iron, then you can add essential oils to both the washing machine and the dryer. Some people choose to add the essential oils to the wash, via the same place they add the washing liquid. I prefer to add the essential oils to one of the items going into the wash. If you do this, make sure that you add it to a part of the item that isn't going to be visible, in case the essential oils damage the fabric. (Do not add oils directly onto delicate items.) If you want to add essential oils to the dryer, try adding them to a disposable cloth used to add fabric conditioner to the load, or add the essential oils to a clean dishcloth.

These essential oils are particularly lovely in the iron: neroli, lavender, rose, rosewood, pine, geranium. Using cedarwood will repel moths.

These are good in the dryer or the washing machine: lavender, rosewood, lemongrass, palmarosa, lemon. (Use citrus oils in small doses as they may sometimes stain.)

FAQs — About blending

Will putting essential oils in my iron damage it?

No, as long as you use the essential oils that are not resinous (avoid benzoin, for instance) and that you don't apply them directly to a hot iron.

What bath products can I make for my baby? She is nine months old and a very erratic sleeper.

As your child is under one year old, you need to be very careful of the amounts of essential oil you use in anything you make for her. Try vaporising essential oils in her room first (lavender, Roman chamomile, mandarin or benzoin are all very useful). If this doesn't help, try putting one drop of lavender and one drop of chamomile in 100 ml of bubble bath (the type of fragrance-free bubble bath specially designed for babies). You may also find that it would be more effective to develop the habit of giving your baby a massage after her bath in order to encourage her to sleep better. The ritual that seems to work best is bath, massage, bottle (or breast), bed. Try doing everything from the massage onwards in dim lighting as this will also encourage sleep.

I want to create a mild scrub for my face, what can you suggest?

Be careful about how often you use a scrub on your face. Most of us seem to think that we need to exfoliate the face regularly in order to get a fresh-seeming complexion, when the reverse is generally true (an enriching masque and the appropriate use of cleansers, facial oils and moisturisers will usually be more effective, even on oily skin). If you still feel you need a facial scrub, then a very gentle one would involve adding 1 teaspoon of ground almonds (available in the baking section of most supermarkets) to 20 ml of cleansing lotion. Please do not use sugar or salt as a scrub on the face as both of these products are too harsh for this delicate area.

What can I do to fragrance my car?

You can get a small vaporiser for your car that plugs in to the cigarette lighter. These are available through many high street outlets.

aromatherapy
massage routine

This chapter contains a suggested routine for a full body massage. If you are planning on including a treatment of the face, it is best to start with the face, then move on to the rest of the body, finishing with the back. This ensures that you are working as hygienically as possible. If your friend does not want a facial treatment, then try starting the treatment from the back (do everything in reverse order), finishing off with the neck and shoulders.

Before you start the treatment, remember to clean the feet (use antiseptic wipes) and wash your hands.

If you do all the movements listed here, you can expect the routine to take you from one to one and a half hours. Shorten it by leaving sections out. With practice, you can do a back, neck and shoulders treatment in half an hour.

Order of treatment:

Face – Neck & Shoulders – Left arm – Left leg – Right leg – Right arm – Abdomen – Roll the client over – Left leg – Right Leg – Back – Finish

The Face

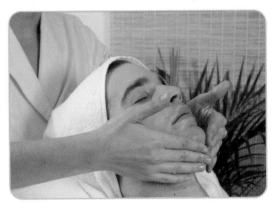

1 Apply oil to face

53

aromatherapy in essence

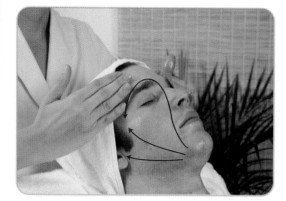

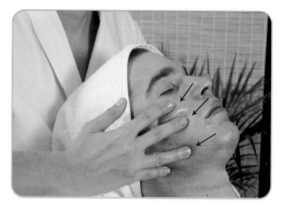

2 Effleurage the face. Keep this rhythmic, gentle and flowing from chin to ears, chin to temples and then from the chin, around the mouth, up the sides of the nose and across the forehead. Return to the chin and repeat the movement. Repeat effleurage after each of the following movements if you want to lengthen the duration of the massage

4 Raking movement to lower part of the face, moving fingers towards the ears

5 Using fingertips, circular stroking around mouth and then over the muscles of the lower face and jawline. If you feel the muscles are tense, you can increase the pressure slightly

6 Massage ears

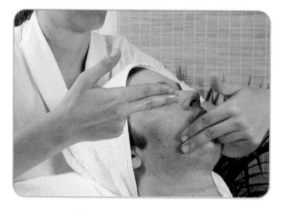

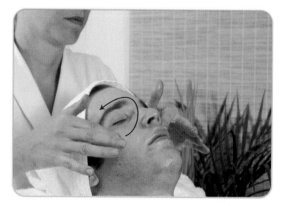

3 Tapotement – Using two fingers from each hand pat along the jawline, then in lines across the lower face working up to the cheekbones

7 Circular strokes around eyes, taking movements out towards the temples

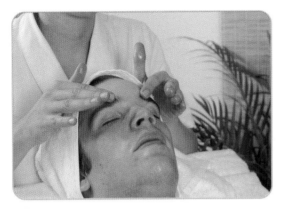

8 Gentle pressure along the eyebrow, take the movement to the temples and rotate gently

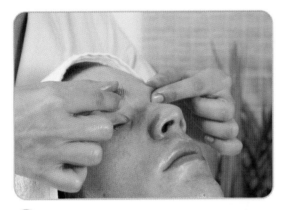

9 Pinch out along eyebrow from inner brow, stroke to temple

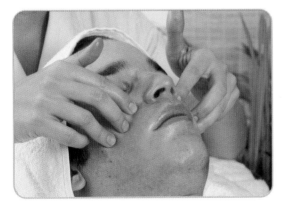

10 Apply gentle pressures over sinuses, around eyebrows and under cheekbones

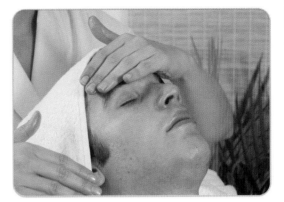

11 Alternate stroking with palm over forehead

12 Effleurage to finish.

Neck and Shoulders (face up)

1 Expose neck and shoulders, apply oil to upper chest, shoulders and back of neck using slow smooth (effleurage) strokes

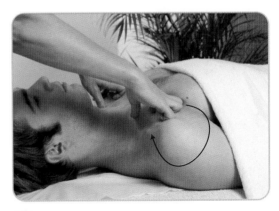

2 Knuckling to shoulders, upper chest and back (don't go below the third rib, this can be very painful, especially if the person you are massaging has large or painful breasts)

55

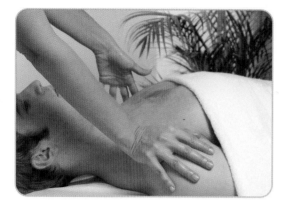

3 Stretching out to pectoral muscles (place your hands on each shoulder and lean first on one shoulder then on the next in a see-saw motion)

4 Slow circular grinding (petrissage) movements (using your thumbs) to the tops of the shoulder and the muscles of the upper back. Movements should be in small circles, then in straight lines, starting from the root of the neck and moving outwards towards the shoulder

5 Repeat effleurage to the back of the neck, stretching the muscles slightly by gently leaning back each time your hands come to the skull

Arms

1 Expose arm. Apply oil over entire arm and shoulder in smooth flowing (effleurage) movements

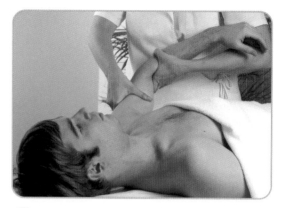

2 Kneading to the whole arm, you may find it easier to lift the elbow and knead the upper arm with just one hand

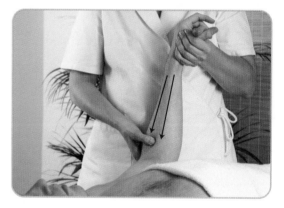

3 Drainage to forearm – raise forearm to the vertical position, use your thumb to drain in straight lines from the wrist to the elbow. Then lift the elbow and repeat the movement for the upper arm

4 Double handed drainage around the shoulder – cup the shoulder between your hands and rub your hands back and forth over the joint in a sawing movement

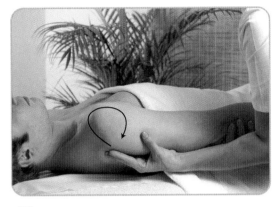

5 Passive rotation to the shoulder – grasp the upper arm in one hand and the elbow with the other, lifting and rotating the shoulder in a 'shrugging movement'

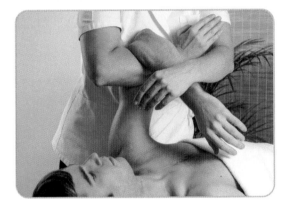

6 Passive stretch to the shoulder – raise the arm, folding the forearm over your arm and by standing on your toes you will lift the arm away from the massage couch, allowing for a passive stretch to the back and shoulder muscles

7 Effleurage of the hand

8 Finger frictions between the bones of the hand

9 Use your thumbs to make small grinding (petrissage) movements to the arm and wrist area

10 Extend the grinding movements over each finger, gently stretching to the joints

11 Effleurage strokes to the whole arm to finish

Legs (face up)

1 Expose the leg and apply oil in smooth strokes over the entire surface of the leg

2 Effleurage × 3 strokes of each of the following
a. Hands opposing

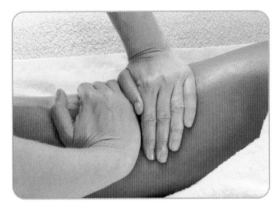

b. Hand leading hand

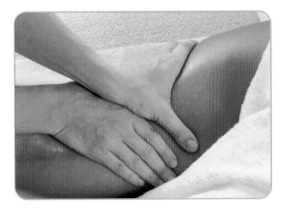

3 Kneading to the thigh area

4 Knuckling to thigh area

5 Deep heel of hand drainage to outer thigh

6 Finger frictions (fast circles) around the knee and repeat for the ankle

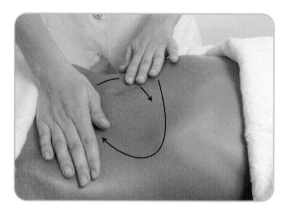

2 Circular effleurage

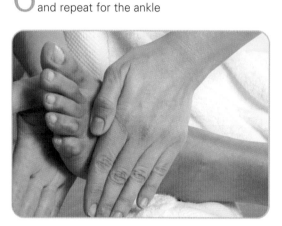

7 Vertical effleurage to the foot

8 Deep pressures to base of the foot – first with your fingers in five strips down from toes to heel, then using your fist into instep

9 Repeat effleurage, gradually becoming lighter to finish

(Repeat for right leg)

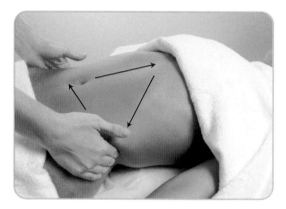

3 Lateralising effleurage

Abdomen

1 Expose belly to ribcage and down to hips, apply oil

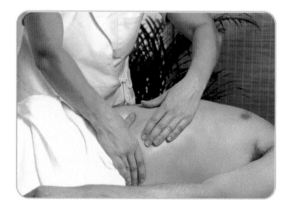

4 Kneading to waist area – first on opposite side and then the side closest to where you are standing

5 Repeat circular effleurage

B: Legs (face down)

1 Expose the leg and apply oil

2 Effleurage × 3 strokes of each of the following
   a. Hands opposing
   b. Hand leading hand

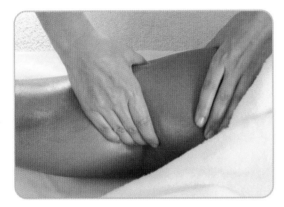

3 Kneading to whole of thigh area, repeat for the calf area

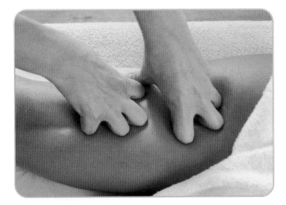

4 Knuckling to thigh area

5 Lymphatic drainage to thigh area – press in hard with your thumbs in three deep lines along the middle of the thigh and towards each side (if they have any cellulite you will feel as if you are 'popping' bubble wrap)

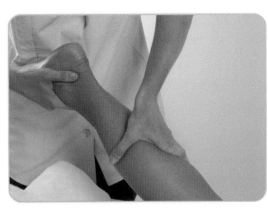

6 Lymph drainage to lower leg – raise the lower leg to allow gravity to assist you. Work in three strips along the calf muscles

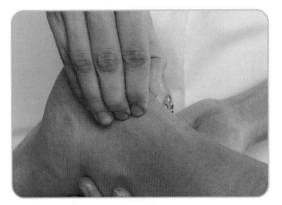

7 Use fingers and thumbs to provide frictions (small circular movements) to the back of the heel.

8 Repeat effleurage

9 Repeat for other leg

Back

1 Standing to the person's left, expose the back and upper buttocks and apply oil.

2 Standard effleurage up the back from the hips to the top of the shoulders, returning along the sides of the body

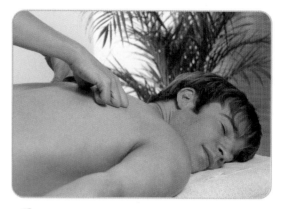

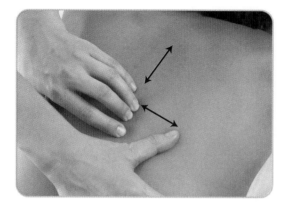

3 Fountain effleurage

4 Kneading over the entire back starting with the opposite side of the body, from hips to shoulder, across shoulders, and then down to the left side of the body from shoulder to hips

6 Knuckling over entire back, concentrating on areas of tension, particularly around the upper back.

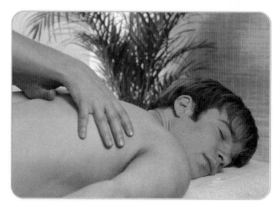

7 Petrissage over the muscles lying to either side of the spine (erector spinae) and over any other areas of tension

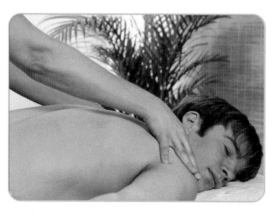

5 Repeat standard effleurage

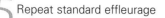

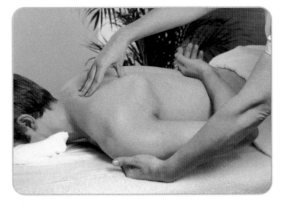

8 Working with the arm closest to you, place the person's wrist into the small of their back, getting them to drop their elbow so that the inner edge of the shoulder blades rises, exposing the underlying muscle. Petrissage to the area.

9 Repeat effleurage and kneading over the entire back.

10 Reinforce hands – circular effleurage to opposite buttock

11 Kneading to opposite buttock

12 Heel of hand stretching to opposite buttock

13 Repeat kneading to side of the body, moving up to the top of the couch

14 Petrissage to upper trapezius from top of the couch

15 Walk to the other side of the body and repeat steps 4–12

16 Repeat petrissage to erector spinae

17 Standard effleurage of whole of the back, movements get lighter as you slow to finish

aromatherapy massage routine

FAQs – About massage

How important is it to always do the massage in the same order?

It isn't important. As you get more experienced, you'll feel more comfortable about adapting what you know to suit the person you are working on. For example, if they are very anxious or stressed you could try working on the face as many find this the most relaxing part of the treatment. If you have someone who has never had massage before try working on their back first as it may take a while for them to feel comfortable with your touch.

I read somewhere that aromatherapy massage is lighter than normal massage. Is this true?

It doesn't have to be. Generally, aroma-therapists will avoid using percussion strokes (like hacking or cupping) in a treatment, although these might well be employed if the therapist was doing a cellulite treatment. However, the other massage strokes you use can be as firm and therapeutic as both you and your client desire.

How much oil should I apply?

You need to get a good 'slip' – so that the area you are working on is covered and your hands can move without friction over the entire surface (and yet it shouldn't be so slippery that your hands slide off). If you pour the oil into the centre of your palm, start with the same amount that, if it were shampoo, you would use to wash your hair. You can always reapply if the person's skin absorbs the oil too fast.

How important is it that I maintain contact with the body I am working on throughout the treatment?

Maintaining contact helps to keep the massage flowing smoothly and will aid relaxation. It will also help you to concentrate on the treatment. Maintaining contact doesn't have to be difficult, but you might want to consider how you have arranged your space before you start. Keep the bottle of oil within reach at all times, if you have notes for your routine (or you are using this book), prop them where you can read them. Also, if you have to check your notes, keep effleuraging your partner while you read them; don't lift your hands off completely.

Aromatherapy in practice

Giving an aromatherapy treatment involves pulling together everything you have learned so far and putting it into practice.

Whilst the magic and the creativity of aromatherapy might be in the blending, the care and the therapeutic value of the massage application in particular cannot be underestimated. Yes, essential oils can enhance a massage, but you need a good, thorough massage routine in order for the treatment to be both enjoyable and therapeutic.

the face and skin

Using essential oils to treat the face and skin is one of the most enjoyable areas of aromatherapy. It is also easy to develop aromatherapy facial treatments for yourself. Remember that if you are treating a particular skin condition it will usually take about 3–4 weeks to reap the benefits of your hard work. This is because the epidermis (the top layer of the skin) takes roughly 21 days to completely regenerate – exactly the amount of time it takes your tan to fade after you return from a holiday. This chapter looks at the different skin types and suggests aromatherapy treatments for the skin.

Simple skin analysis

To treat the skin effectively, you need to have a basic idea of how to identify the different skin types. You will need to examine the skin in bright light, when the person is not wearing makeup.

The different types of skin fall into the following categories:

- oily
- combination
- normal
- sensitive
- mature/sun-damaged skin
- dry skin
- dehydrated skin
- acne rosacea
- acne vulgaris.

Oily skin

Identified by its shiny appearance (although it dries out with age), oily skin tends to be thicker and coarser than other skin types and is usually less sensitive. There is a tendency for blackheads, whiteheads, clogged pores and other blemishes. Essential oils that are especially useful here are those that balance hormonal activity and the production of sebum and those that are antiseptic. Try cedarwood, lavender, geranium, ylang ylang, peppermint, juniper, orange, cypress, lemon, clary sage, tea tree, rosewood, sandalwood, rosemary, or bergamot.

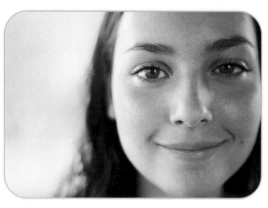

An oily skin

Combination skin

Combination skin can be either normal/dry or normal/oily. There is a distinctly different structure and appearance to the skin between the T-zone and the rest of the face. Pores around the nose will be larger than elsewhere and there will be distinct areas of the face which are shiny or matte. Where breakouts occur, these are usually linked to hormonal fluctuations. Try geranium, lavender, neroli, rosewood, sandalwood, ylang ylang, or palmarosa.

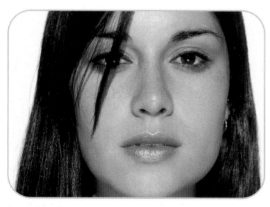

A combination skin

Normal skin

There is some debate over whether the only *really* normal skin is that seen in children. Normal skin is neither too oily nor too dry, has very few blemishes and little or no sun damage. The skin is smooth, firm and appears plump and dewy. People lucky enough to have normal skin are advised to continue with what they are doing and treat their skin with any essential oils that are designed to provide emotional support or to treat other presenting issues. Try lavender, jasmine, ylang ylang, rosewood, clary sage, geranium, rose, neroli.

Sensitive skin

Sensitive skin is easily irritated. Generally, sensitive skin is thinner than other skin types. Because the nerve endings and blood vessels are so close to the skin's surface, sensitive skin is more likely to react to trigger products and is also more likely to react adversely to essential oils. There are three main causes of sensitive skin: stress, environmental factors and hormonal activity.

Stress-related sensitive skin is sensitive to emotional turmoil and worsened by stress. Acne will develop when the person is stressed and is particularly likely to develop where frequent air travel is a feature of the person's life. Any breakout is made worse by the person touching their skin. Choose essential oils that address any other symptoms of stress the person is experiencing and also try Roman chamomile, lavender, rose, geranium, ylang ylang.

Skin that is sensitive to environmental factors tends to develop allergic reactions: to food, beauty products or cleaning products. It is easily irritated, especially if products are overused. This person is also prone to insect attack (they may joke about being the best person to sit next to at a picnic) and the chances are that they will be very sensitive to essential oils. Choose oils that are very gentle and not prone to causing sensitisation: Roman chamomile, geranium, jasmine – but patch testing is recommended, lavender, patchouli, rose, rosewood, sandalwood, cedarwood, ylang ylang.

Skin that is sensitive due to hormonal activity tends to break out before menstrual periods, is made worse by the use of any oral contraceptives or steroid drugs and tends to be sensitive to the weather. Try essential oils that are known to regulate hormonal activity, as well as anti-anxiety products: geranium, jasmine, fennel, clary sage, orange, neroli, sandalwoood, patchouli, yarrow, German chamomile, Roman chamomile, rosewood, lavender.

Mature/sun-damaged skin

It is sometimes assumed that the skin of all those who are over a certain age will exhibit the symptoms of mature skin. This is not the case. People in their twenties who overuse the sunbed or who have been exposed to the elements for extended periods of time are likely to show early signs of damage. Older people who have taken care of their skin and their health are likely to have good skin that belies their years. Neglected skin may be recognised by a distinct leathery texture, visible wrinkles, dull skin, age spots (or large freckles) on the face, hands, back or feet. A loss of skin tone around the cheeks and jawline and the tendency for the skin to feel dry and tight, especially in cold weather, are also noticeable. With this type of skin, the emphasis is to help the skin regenerate properly, to reduce blotchiness and thread veins and to help to balance sebum production. Try using: neroli, lavender, frankincense, ylang ylang, geranium, carrot seed, Roman chamomile, rose, yarrow, German chamomile, clary sage, patchouli, cypress, rosewood, sandalwood, immortelle, myrrh.

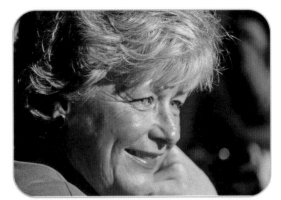

Mature skin

Dry skin

Dry skin can be differentiated from dehydrated skin because as well as feeling tight, there is visible flaking of the skin in some areas. It tends to be matte in appearance, sensitive to cold, to wrinkle easily and, occasionally, to feel rough to the touch. Essential oils known for their moisturising properties and their ability to encourage sebum production include: lavender, sandalwood, geranium, rose, neroli, Roman chamomile, clary sage, jasmine, patchouli, rosewood, sandalwood, ylang ylang, German chamomile, palmarosa.

Dehydrated

This skin type simply lacks water. There may be fine lines, so it is often mistaken for dry skin. However, there will also be evidence of other types of skin (clogged pores and blackheads, for instance). Reddening, dryness or flaking around the nostrils, broken blood vessels or a chapped appearance are the key indicators to look for. As well as increasing water intake, use essential oils that help to heal the skin and balance out any sebum production: frankincense, benzoin, geranium, lavender, neroli, patchouli, rose, sandalwood.

Acne rosacea

This form of acne tends to develop in a person's late twenties and is most easily identified by the distinctive redness brought on by broken capillaries on the cheeks, nose and forehead.

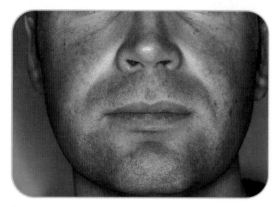

Acne rosacea

Unlike acne vulgaris, any lesions appear as red bumps (almost as though the acne is under the skin, rather than on top of it), or a persistent redness to the facial area. It will not respond to the usual acne treatments. Nasal bumps will occur, especially in men, which contributes to an appearance of swollen nose and cheeks. Avoid any essential oils that are designed to increase circulation. Use anti-inflammatories and vein tonics to reduce any broken blood vessels or visible capillaries. Try Roman chamomile, cypress, German chamomile, yarrow, palmarosa, neroli, lavender.

Acne vulgaris

This is the type of acne that we associate with teenagers, although they certainly don't have a monopoly on the condition. The pustular eruptions respond best to essential oils that have skin healing properties, are antiseptic, antibiotic and will heal wounds. Try lavender, geranium, juniper, tea tree, rosewood, Roman chamomile, sandalwood, cedarwood, clary sage, frankincense, immortelle, ylang ylang.

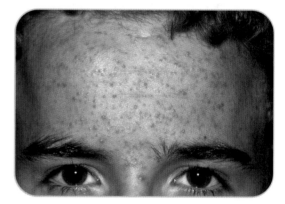

Acne vulgaris

Creating an aromatherapy facial experience

For a completely exotic and luxurious experience, use this routine, which includes cleansing, toning, a facial mask and the facial massage. You can carry out this routine on yourself or on a friend. Follow these steps:

1 Cleanse the skin. Use dampened make up pads (or cotton balls) to apply an aromatherapy cleanser you have created. If the skin is very blotchy, or if the person is wearing

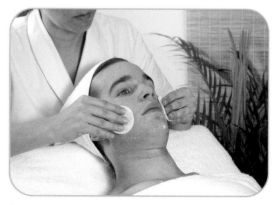

Cleansing the skin

makeup, cleanse twice. If there is any beard growth, you may find it easier to apply cleanser with a flannel rather than cotton wool, which will get stuck in facial hair.

2 Tone the skin. Starting with dry makeup pads, use toner to dampen the pads, then pat them over the face, paying particular attention to any blemished areas or where pores are visibly larger.

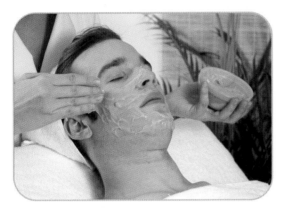

Facial mask

3 Apply a face mask. You may like to try one of the recipes on the next few pages. The following food masks have all been tried and tested and generally smell good enough to eat! For the most part, they are enriching masks. If the skin is very blemished, you may want to try a natural yoghurt mask instead. Remove the masks with warm water, pat the skin dry and, if necessary, cleanse again.

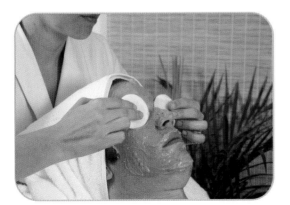

Under-eye pads

4 Apply the under-eye treatment. Use make-up pads dampened with the treatment material. Place these over the closed eyes while the mask is on.

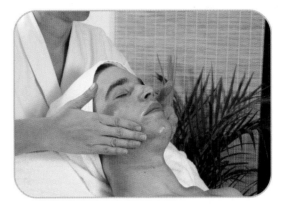

Applying facial oil

5 Apply a facial oil blend. Use gentle and flowing movements from chin to ears, chin to temples, then from the chin, around the mouth, up the sides of the nose and across the forehead. Return to the chin and repeat the movement. You will probably need to use between 5 and 10 ml of facial oil. If the skin is very dry and the facial oil is completely absorbed, add a moisturiser at the end of the treatment to seal in the treatment oils.

The treatment may take between 20 minutes and an hour, depending on how often you repeat the individual massage strokes.

Note: Remember, keep the blends simple and don't use too many essential oils on the face. Never apply face masks to the eye area unless it is a specified recipe for the eyes.

Try this:

To help combination skin that is currently dehydrated (perhaps as a result of stress and lack of sleep):

- Cleanser – 1 drop of rosewood in 20 ml of cleanser
- Toner – rosewater hydrolat
- Mask – avocado (applied outside the T-zone), savoury mask (applied on the T-zone)
- Under-eye treatment – papaya juice
- Facial oil – sandalwood, neroli, rosewood (1 drop each) in 20 ml of jojoba oil.

To cleanse very oily or acne-ridden skin:

- lemon – 3 drops
- juniper – 1 drop
- lavender – 4 drops

in 40 ml of cleanser.

Facial oil to reduce the appearance of wrinkles:

- frankincense – 2 drops
- sandalwood – 1 drop
- rose –1 drop

in 20 ml of avocado or argan oil.

To reduce enlarged pores (use one drop of one of these essential oils in the toner, and this recipe for the facial oil):

- grapefruit 1 drop
- peppermint 1 drop
- cypress 2 drops

in 20 ml of calendula (or hazelnut) oil.

To reduce the appearance of broken capillaries:

- cypress – 2 drops
- bergamot – 1 drop
- patchouli – 1 drop

in 20 ml of jojoba oil.

Face mask recipes

Banana mask

This mask is great for dry, dehydrated or mature skin. Purée a whole banana (riper bananas will have a deeper cleansing effect). Leave on for no more than ten minutes.

Coconut and honey mask

This smells absolutely fantastic. You can use either coconut milk (tinned or in cartons) or coconut cream. The cream gets you a thicker consistency, which is more useful if you want to move around while the mask is on. If using coconut milk, use 50 ml of milk to one tablespoon of thick honey, mix well, leave on for ten minutes. If using coconut cream, mix 10 g of coconut cream with one tablespoon of honey and add warm water until you get the desired consistency. Leave on for between five and ten minutes.

Papaya mask

This is useful for normal or combination skin, especially if it has been under some stress and there are dark circles under the eyes. Purée half a medium-sized ripe papaya. Thicken with aloe vera gel, honey or egg white if necessary.

Strawberry mask

This is good for oily skin, as the strawberries are quite astringent. Remember to check that the person using this is not allergic to strawberries. Purée a handful of strawberries, apply and wash off after ten minutes.

Peach and honey mask

A lovely blend for oily to combination skin, but the peach needs to be properly ripe. Mix one puréed ripe peach with a teaspoon of honey. Rinse off after five minutes.

Avocado mask

A favourite. As well as having an interestingly lurid colour, this is easy to apply and wash off and leaves the skin feeling very smooth, soft and elastic. Purée half a ripe avocado. Add a small amount of water (1–2 tbs) to get a smooth consistency. Leave on for at least five minutes.

Aloe and honey mask

This is very useful where there is inflamed skin that is also infected. Use equal portions of aloe vera gel and runny honey. Use Manuka honey if there are any skin infections or acne.

Green grape mask

This is wonderful for sensitive and oily skins, or for acne. Purée a handful of green grapes. Apply to the skin and leave on for at least ten minutes.

Milk and apple mask

Very useful for sensitive skins, especially due to hormonal activity. Stew an apple gently in full fat milk. Purée it, add a teaspoon honey and leave to cool slightly. Apply when it is still warm, but not hot. Leave on for five minutes.

Savoury mask

Use a medium-sized potato and half cook it in the microwave (put it on for half the amount of time you would when cooking for eating). Purée it in the blender with two heaped tablespoons of yoghurt, sour cream or crème fraîche. This is wonderful if you feel your skin looks dull, needs some detoxifying, or has occasional spots. Leave on for between five and ten minutes.

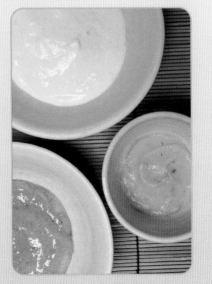

Savoury, avocado and banana masks

Natural under-eye treatments

Ingredient	Effects
Cold teabags	Reduces puffiness, constricts small blood vessels. Very useful when eyes are red from late nights or crying.
Sliced cucumber	Reduces puffiness, mildly detoxifies, constricts small blood vessels. Eyes usually look brighter afterwards.
Aloe vera gel	An anti-inflammatory product which reduces puffiness. Very useful for puffy eyes as a result of hay fever.
Papaya juice	Reduces puffiness and gets rid of dark circles.
Hydrolat (e.g. rose water)	Reduces puffiness.
Raw potato juice (made in juicer)	More astringent than the papaya juice, so works best on oily or normal skin. Reduces puffiness and dark circles.

casestudy: Stress-related acne vulgaris

Frank's acne was clearly stress-related. He mentioned that he was stressed at work, and the acne was concentrated in the beard area (lower face and neck) – a classic presentation of stress-related acne. Before he tried aromatherapy, he was contemplating growing a full beard to cover the spots, despite being a very fashion-conscious 28-year-old.

Treating Frank involved a back, neck and shoulder massage (to help with the stress) as well as a detailed facial treatment and a treatment cleanser and facial oil to use daily between treatments. Four treatment sessions were recommended, at intervals of ten days. Although he initially balked at the idea of using oil on his face, Frank did persevere and was so pleased with the changes he saw in just the first week, that he continues to use oil as a moisturiser even now that his acne has gone.

The initial facial treatment used for Frank involved the following:

- ☊ Green grape mask (see recipe on page 71).
- ☊ Cleanser – sandalwood 1 drop, tea tree 1 drop, in 20 ml of cleanser.
- ☊ Toner – lavender hydrolat (Frank didn't like the smell of this, so we only used it in the treatment sessions, not between sessions).
- ☊ Facial oil – sandalwood 2 drops, tea tree 1 drop, rosewood 2 drops in 30 ml of jojoba. (This oil was also used for the back massage given for use in between sessions).

Although he enjoyed the blends and was very impressed with the effects of the green grape mask, Frank really didn't like using tea tree as he felt it smelled too medicinal and made him all the more aware of the 'problem' his skin had become. As a result, we started experimenting with other anti-bacterial essential oils that are particularly effective at clearing the skin and which he felt smelled more appealing. The treatment blend he was happiest with involved the following:

- Cleanser – juniper 1 drop, sandalwood 1 drop, in 20 ml of cleanser.
- Facial oil – juniper 1 drop, sandalwood 2 drops. bergamot 2 drops, in 30 ml of carrier oil.

Please note that these facial blends are far more dilute than the body blends that are recommended elsewhere in this book.

FAQs – About treating the face and skin

I want to create a moisturising product that will also help to sort out ingrown hairs. It needs to be dual purpose – my boyfriend wants to use it on his beard area and I'd quite like something that is sensitive enough to use on my bikini line after waxing.

Try rosewood (3 drops), tea tree (2 drops) and lavender (3 drops) in 60 ml of unperfumed moisturising cream. This is particularly dilute because you are suggesting using it after waxing. All three essential oils are gentle antiseptics but if you have sensitive skin or you have reacted to products in the past, please wait at least three days after waxing to use this product.

How long will it take before I see an improvement in my skin?

It takes your epidermis (the top layer of your skin) 21 days to regenerate completely. If you persevere with using aromatherapy products, you can expect to see noticeable changes within four weeks.

Can I put make up on over the facial oil?

Yes, although it is best to wait about 15 minutes before you do so. This allows the facial oil to sink into your skin. Jojoba is a very effective carrier oil to use in this way.

I think I have *acne rosacea* and I've tried using calendula oil to clear the acne scars, but it just doesn't seem to agree with my skin. Can you suggest something else?

You would probably respond better to argan, camellia or jojoba oils as a carrier oil. Have a look at the essential oils that you are using, too. Get rid of anything that brings blood to the surface of the skin. Try using lavender, cypress and geranium (3 drops lavender, 3 drops cypress and 2 drops geranium, in 40 ml of carrier oil).

the heart and circulation

At the centre of our cardiovascular systems lies the heart, the hardest-working muscle in the body. Continuously beating from shortly after conception, it has a great deal of physical work to do (and that's before we consider the emotional heartaches that we all experience during our life time). Both massage and aromatherapy have a noticeable effect on the cardiovascular system. The correct use of essential oils and massage can improve the circulation – so blood is moved to and from the body tissues faster and more effectively. The oils can help to clear waste products by encouraging effective detoxification of the tissues. Some oils are known to raise and lower blood pressure, as well as to constrict and dilate the blood vessels.

How the system works

To understand how aromatherapy can help the heart, you need a basic idea of how the cardiovascular system works and some of the terminology associated with it. Blood pressure (BP) is defined as the pressure that the blood exerts on the walls of the arteries as they leave the heart. In an average adult, blood pressure is usually around 120/80 (the top number indicates how much pressure is exerted during systole, the contraction phase of the heart; the bottom number shows how much pressure is exerted during diastole, when the heart is relaxed and is filling up with blood). The force of blood flow is strongest nearest the heart. As the blood vessels get further away from the heart (towards the skin and tissues of, for example the fingers and toes), they get smaller. The pressure drops in the tiny capillaries, so that they remain undamaged. Where blood pressure is raised, or if damage occurs to these capillaries, there may be thread veins, bruising, or the distinctive reddening of broken capillaries. When blood makes its way back from the capillaries to the heart, there is no pump action to help move it back up the body. The only thing helping the movement is the contraction of the muscles in the area. Gravity sometimes encourages blood or lymph to pool in certain areas, usually around the ankles. This can cause muscles in the walls of the veins to stretch and grow slack, which is how varicose veins develop. Massage helps to encourage venous flow – the flow of blood through the veins back to the heart. When used in conjunction with essential oils that help to improve circulation, massage can make a real difference to the health of the cardiovascular system.

Oils to improve circulation: May chang, peppermint, juniper, nutmeg, Atlas cedarwood, ginger, rosemary, black pepper.

Heart palpitations

Heart palpitations, where the heart beats irregularly and too frequently, can feel very uncomfortable and may be frightening if they go on for an extended length of time. Tachycardia, sometimes called palpitations, can be a symptom of more serious conditions, not least that medication you are currently taking does not agree with you. Ylang ylang will help to ease palpitations, but if you are experiencing them regularly it is advised that you discuss it with your doctor.

High blood pressure

Also referred to as hypertension, high blood pressure is when the pressure rises above 175/100. It can be caused by a number of things. The most common reasons include increasing age, lack of exercise, sudden weight gain, high levels of stress and a poor diet (especially if it is high in fat and salt). People can also have a genetic predisposition to raised blood pressure (so if other members of your family have it, you might have it too). Smoking, drinking alcohol regularly and

drinking a lot of caffeine also contribute to raised blood pressure. Reducing the blood pressure takes a lot of time. Studies carried out in the 1990s into the effects of alcohol on the blood pressure showed that while there was some initial improvement in the blood pressure as the individual abstained, it took at least three months of not drinking alcohol before the blood pressure showed any significant and sustained decrease. Aromatherapy can help lower blood pressure, but to be effective at doing so, regular aromatherapy massage *and* other lifestyle changes such as decreasing alcohol, caffeine and nicotine intake and starting to exercise gently but regularly would be necessary.

Essential oils that are particularly useful at helping to lower blood pressure include: clary sage, lavender, marjoram, Roman and German chamomile, valerian, vetiver, spikenard, orange, neroli and ylang ylang.

To lower blood pressure:

- marjoram 2 drops
- lavender 3 drops
- ylang ylang 3 drops

in 20 ml of carrier oil.

Low blood pressure

Low blood pressure, or hypotension, is often regarded as desirable, especially as your blood pressure tends to rise with age. Hypotension is defined as anything less than 100/70. Low blood pressure is only really worrying if it is dropping suddenly, as this usually means that the person is bleeding internally or losing blood rapidly. If someone generally has low blood pressure, then you can expect them to complain about frequently feeling cold, that they sometimes feel dizzy, nauseous or will faint if they get up suddenly. When massaging someone who has low blood pressure it is important to help them to sit up slowly after treatment and wait a few minutes before standing, as massage will reduce the blood pressure anyway. It also means that using essential oils that are known to lower blood pressure is really not a good idea, unless you blend them with other essential oils that will raise blood pressure. Essential oils that raise blood pressure include: rosemary, peppermint and black pepper. Cypress is a vasoconstrictor, so it will also help to raise blood pressure in a small way.

To raise blood pressure:

- cypress 3 drops
- rosemary 2 drops
- lavender 3 drops

in 20 ml of carrier oil.

To balance blood pressure (for the person with low blood pressure who loves ylang ylang):

- ylang ylang 2 drops
- black pepper 3 drops
- grapefruit 3 drops

in 20 ml of carrier oil.

Bruises

A bruise is the visible indication that bleeding has occurred following damage to some of the small blood vessels in the area. It is not recommended that you massage over bruises, not least because it will be painful. However, cold compresses can help to ease the pain, reduce the swelling and heal the tissues. Lavender, ginger, peppermint or cypress are all helpful in these cases.

When a person presents with bruises and they 'don't know how they did it', they may be someone who bruises easily, but there is also the possibility that their mind is dealing with so many things all at once that they aren't really aware of what is going on for their body. Vetiver is considered to be one of the most effective 'grounding' essential oils. Try this blend as a massage oil and use it elsewhere on the body (not over the bruises themselves):

- vetiver 3 drops
- ginger 2 drops
- geranium 3 drops

in 20 ml of carrier oil.

Reynaud's syndrome

Reynaud's syndrome is an interesting condition that features poor circulation as a major symptom. The tiny capillaries that feed the cells and tissues around the body all branch off from different arteries. At the start of each network of capillaries, there is a sphincter muscle that will open or close depending on the needs of the body. So, for example, when you are in the process of digesting a meal the sphincter muscles around the blood vessels near your stomach and intestines will open up, so that the plentiful blood supply to this area can absorb all the nutrients of your meal. In cold weather, the sphincter muscles around the capillary networks feeding the peripheral areas (your hands, feet and skin) will close down so that blood to these areas is limited and stays in the central areas of your body to keep warm. In someone with Reynaud's syndrome, something has gone wrong with the sphincter muscles around the capillaries in their hands and feet, so they tend to have very poor circulation to these areas, even when the body is warm elsewhere. They will complain about the cold and also about the pain associated with the blood going back to these areas. What is interesting to observe is that while there can be a family predisposition to this condition, it is often connected with stress, so with treatment for poor circulation and stress the results are better. Try this as a blend:

- black pepper 4 drops
- rosemary 1 drop
- neroli (or rose) 3 drops

in 20 ml of carrier oil (for massage).

This can also be used as a moisturiser on the hands and feet between treatments.

Varicose veins

Varicose veins develop where the veins become distended as there is too much blood (or lymph) pooling in the area (usually in the

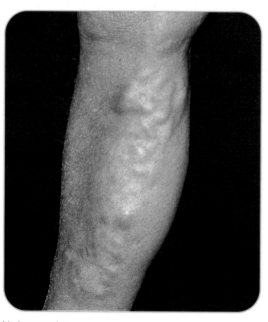

Varicose veins

lower legs). Raising the legs can make a big difference to the comfort of the person, as can gentle massage. Massage should only be above the area and encourage blood flow back to the heart, and *never* over the veins themselves as they are very fragile. Before you use the blend suggested herewith, remember to take into consideration the circumstances that led to the development of the varicose veins as this may affect your choice of essential oils. This condition can arise out of a family history of varicose veins, from pregnancy, sudden weight gain, or standing for long periods of time. If pregnancy is involved, you will need to adjust the strength of the blend. If there has been weight gain, you may want to think about how desirable it might be to look at detoxing and possibly losing some weight. Where the person has to stand for a long time, you may want to consider essential oils to help relieve muscle pain too – try black pepper or lemongrass with cypress in these cases. Another activity that can really help to improve the condition of the veins on the lower legs is to use hot and cold water over them. In the shower, alternate between hot and cold water for 30 seconds at a time and repeat for up to two minutes daily. Try this blend:

- lemon 2 drops
- cypress 4 drops
- neroli 2 drops

in 20 ml of carrier oil.

casestudy: Dealing with high blood pressure

Roger had recently been diagnosed as having high blood pressure. It had reached a point where his doctor was considering putting him on medication for high blood pressure (it was 185/105). Roger asked the doctor if it would be possible for him to try to control his blood pressure by using complementary and alternative treatments first. His doctor agreed that Roger could go ahead, on condition that he returned within three months to have his blood pressure monitored and that if he started getting headaches regularly or feeling under the weather he was to come back immediately, regardless of whether he thought he might be wasting the doctor's time. He was also told to stop smoking, to cut salt out of his diet and to halve his alcohol intake.

Roger did all of this, although he found giving up the cigarettes particularly difficult. He compromised on his alcohol intake by making sure that he used the units he was 'allowed' for special occasions and where he could really enjoy his drink without feeling guilty (and without binge-drinking). He also bought a blood pressure measuring cuff, so he could monitor his own blood pressure to see how it changed.

Because Roger needed very regular treatment to help reduce his blood pressure, it was decided that the most effective way of using aromatherapy for him would be if his partner gave him a short massage twice daily (at the start of the day, immediately after waking, so that he remained calm throughout the day and again at the end of the evening, in order to unwind). When his partner was not able to massage him, he was to have a warm (not hot), bath with the appropriate blend in it.

Two of the most effective essential oils for high blood pressure are clary sage and ylang ylang. Although Roger wasn't fond of either essential oil, he found them acceptable in the following blends.

For use any time:
- clary sage 2 drops
- ylang ylang 2 drops
- juniper 4 drops

in 20 ml carrier oil.

cont.

For evening use:
- clary sage 2 drops
- vetiver 3 drops
- rosewood 3 drops

in 20 ml carrier oil.

For daytime use:
- ylang ylang 3 drops
- lavender 2 drops
- lemon 3 drops

in 20 ml of carrier oil.

Roger started taking his blood pressure before and after each treatment. He noted that after three weeks, it had dropped significantly. At the end of three months, he saw his doctor, who was pleased with his progress but did not want to rule out the possibility of giving Roger drugs to reduce his blood pressure at a later date, especially if he returned to his old habits! Roger continues to have his blood pressure monitored every three months (and to have aromatherapy massages at least every other day).

the digestive system

The sense of smell is closely linked to the act of digestion. When you smell food cooking, your mouth probably starts to water in anticipation and your body makes further preparations to digest a meal.

Digestive complaints tend to respond very well to aromatherapy. However, it is not generally advisable to take the essential oils themselves by mouth. There are a few exceptions to this. For example, it is possible to get peppermint oil capsules from some chemists as part of a treatment for irritable bowel syndrome. The peppermint helps to ease the painful muscle spasms that are associated with this condition. (Peppermint and chamomile herbal teas also help.) For many years, dentists have used oil of clove as a remedy for severe toothache (as well as to provide pain relief when filling teeth) and myrrh and tea tree to reduce the effects of gum disease. None of these products taste remotely pleasant and should not be taken by mouth, although they can be useful as a support for these conditions if added in low dilutions to a facial oil and used over the painful areas of the face.

Abdominal massage

A careful massage of the abdominal area using appropriate essential oils can help to ease pain and return the body to its natural state of balance and rhythm. When massaging the abdomen, ensure that you keep your movements slow and rhythmical. Practise on yourself first. The pressure needs to be firm enough to avoid tickling, but not deep. Carry out the massage in a clock-wise direction. You are trying to mimic the effects of peristalsis – the wave-like contractions of the oesophagus, stomach and small intestine that push food along the gastro-intestinal tract. If your friend or relative is uncomfortable about having

81

massage done on their abdomen, they can do it themselves. If practised with care, it will make an enormous difference to their state of health.

Essential oils that are particularly useful in massage for digestive complaints include: black pepper, peppermint, fennel, juniper, thyme, coriander, ginger, grapefruit, marjoram, clove, nutmeg, orange, mandarin, tangerine, rosemary, geranium, myrrh, tea tree, chamomile and cardamom.

Anorexia and bulimia

Conditions such as anorexia and bulimia, while associated with the digestive system, are emotional or psychological conditions and should be treated as such. There are often deeply buried feelings of rage, anger, sorrow, poor body image or self-hatred and self-disgust involved when people experience these conditions. These feelings are expressed through their reactions to food as, in some cases, food is seen as the one thing they can control in their lives. When using aromatherapy the areas to concentrate on are improving feelings of self-worth, increasing appetite (especially for people with anorexia) and encouraging a more balanced approach to coping. Initially, people with bulimia or anorexia may be reluctant to be massaged. If this is the case, see if massages of the hands, face, or feet are acceptable. If you manage to get them to agree to having a full body massage (especially including the abdomen), you will have achieved a great deal. In addition to the essential oils recommended for the digestive system, aromatherapy blends for these conditions benefit greatly from the inclusion of palmarosa (where there is rage and anger, rose (to help with self-hatred), neroli (where

there is anxiety, depression or low self-worth) and fennel (where emotional as well as physical detoxification is indicated).

Constipation

Constipation plagues many of us at some time. Some nutritionists state that a regular bowel habit involves one or two movements a day, but others say that 'regular' means a habit that is normal for you, whether it is one or two movements a day, or a movement every couple of days. When your habits cease to be regular, the discomfort, bloating and feelings of being overly full need to be dealt with as soon as possible. Choose essential oils that are particularly useful for easing muscle spasms and use the blend for a slow abdominal massage. A useful blend is:

- peppermint 3 drops
- geranium 2 drops
- juniper 3 drops

in 20 ml of carrier oil.

In this blend, black pepper can be used instead of peppermint; and fennel instead of juniper.

Diarrhoea

When considering how to treat diarrhoea, it is important to look at the underlying causes. If it is as a result of an infection or food poisoning then using essential oils with antibacterial properties as well as those designed to relieve pain will be most appropriate. Try the following, in a warm compress:

- tea tree 1 drop
- rosewood 1 drop
- ginger 1 drop.

Gum disease

Myrrh and tea tree are the most useful essential oils to treat gum disease, although they are very powerful in combination. If you dislike either of these essential oils try the following in a facial blend designed to relieve pain and inflammation:

- Roman chamomile 1 drop
- nutmeg 1 drop
- lavender 2 drops

in 20 ml of carrier oil.

Loss of appetite

Loss of appetite can be a positive condition if you are trying to lose weight, but when it accompanies more serious symptoms (such as extreme nausea, or depression) it is often vital to improve the appetite if the person is going to be able to return to a balanced state of health. Essential oils which are derived from fruits, foods and spices tend to be particularly useful, especially if they evoke memories in the individual of times where they enjoyed meals or felt comforted. Try orange, lemon, black pepper, rosemary, ginger, tangerine, mandarin, benzoin or peppermint.

Stomach ulcers

Gentle abdominal massage can help to soothe the pain and discomfort of ulcers. Your choice of essential oils for supporting ulcers (and their treatment), will depend on what caused the ulcer to develop. If it is stress-related, then choose essential oils that are indicated for anxiety – such as neroli, clary sage, fennel, peppermint, frankincense, rose or geranium. If the ulcer turns out to be as a result of a bacterial infection (the bacterium *Helicobacter pylori* is believed to be responsible for a wide range of serious conditions, ranging from ulcers right through to heart condition), then using essential oils which have a strong anti-bacterial action is most appropriate. Try tea tree, rosewood, sandalwood, cypress or lavender.

Encouraging weight loss

Just as there is a weight loss diet plan for almost every day of the year, so we can develop a large range of aromatherapy blends that will work to encourage weight loss. The secret to finding a blend that works for you is to be completely honest with yourself about what the underlying reasons for any undesired weight might be. If it is 'winter fat' to keep you warm, then try something that will increase your circulation, like rosemary or black pepper. If it is 'pre-menstrual hunger' which finds you diving head first into the chocolate and sugar, try sweet smelling oils which are also closely linked to the endocrine system, for example, benzoin, geranium, or rose. If you know it is the slow accumulation of years of eating unwisely, try blends of essential oils that are particularly effective at detoxing the system, for example, grapefruit, juniper, fennel or vetiver. Lastly, if you know it is mainly due to a lack of exercise (and a lack of motivation to do anything), try essential oils that will kick-start your motivation – ginger is best for this.

casestudy: Irritable Bowel Syndrome (IBS)

Sangita had been suffering with the symptoms of IBS for four years, following the removal of her appendix in her twenties. The condition can develop following surgery, but Sangita admits that it was likely to have happened at any time given the high stress levels she was under (she worked as a travelling sales representative, did not take regular breaks and ate at her desk or in her car). Sangita experienced her IBS as alternating bouts of constipation and diarrhoea. She tended to have three to four days of constipation, with accompanying bloating and no bowel movements, and would experience the diarrhoea on the morning of the fifth day (on which she would not be bloated) before the cycle returned to constipation. While Sangita had adapted to living with this pattern, she found that the discomfort of the bloating and the associated pain was increasing.

The essential oils that are most relevant to Sangita's particular situation include ginger, peppermint, geranium and black pepper. Of these, the peppermint tends to be the most popular choice as it is not only soothing to nervous digestive systems, but it is also a very effective antispasmodic (which means it stops the muscle spasms that would account for some of the pain Sangita was experiencing).

Sangita loved the peppermint, but did not respond well to the ginger oil despite using ginger frequently in cooking. Through trial and error we arrived at a blend that was particularly effective at supporting Sangita and which (with daily abdominal massage) allowed her to regulate her bowel habits and to produce more 'solid' stools, as well as reducing the pain and bloating. Sangita's favourite blend was: peppermint 4 drops, neroli 2 drops, bergamot 2 drops, in 20 ml of carrier oil.

Sangita found that making some small lifestyle changes was essential to helping her digestive system return to a more balanced state of health. She started drinking herbal teas (chamomile and peppermint), having at least three cups of herbal tea a day in addition to a minimum of two litres of water a day. She also found that reducing the amount of wheat in her diet had a profound effect (though she did not have coeliac disease). When she came for her last treatment, she commented that although not having wheat meant that she couldn't accept biscuits when they were offered to her at meetings, she felt she wasn't suffering too much as her favourite chocolate bars did not contain wheat!

the mind and nervous system

Treating the mind and nervous system is one of the most satisfying areas of working with aromatherapy. Dealing with issues to do with the mind, the emotions, or with nerve-related pain force you to take a more personal approach to the essential oils – one where you are actively searching for the best blend for the person on the day. You may need to go off the beaten track to treat someone effectively: just because there is a list of essential oils that aid anxiety or depression, doesn't mean that the first ones on the list are going to be right for the person being treated. Some choices can be surprising. I met someone who found rosemary completely sedating, whereas normally rosemary isn't used after 4 pm in case it affects sleep. Similarly, cypress is not known for its sedative effects, but if someone is lying awake with their mind in overdrive, it is definitely recommended when blended with other, more sedating oils.

Perhaps the easiest way to help you decide how to treat nervous conditions is to consider them in terms of the pain experienced. Nerve pain, such as sciatica or neuralgia, are fairly easy to approach. Here, you would need strong analgesics, especially those with a close link to the nervous system: basil, valerian, or carrot seed are particularly useful, as are cinnamon, clove or nutmeg although none of them are particularly pleasant to smell unless blended appropriately. (They are also contraindicated in certain situations, so careful checking is necessary.)

Emotional pain, in contrast, is harder to analyse, not least because there may well be reasons for the person to deny that they are feeling any pain at all. Perhaps to admit there are problems is against their principles, it might be that they want to save you (or someone else) from the discomfort of knowing what they are feeling. Admitting the problem may be in conflict with their personal view of themselves, or it may require them to take a stand or take action in a way they don't want to face. The person who is anxious may be faced with choices they don't want to make. The person who is depressed may be unable to do anything (yet mortified to find themselves in this position).

For physical pain, use strong analgesics, including, but not limited to, marjoram, frankincense, black pepper, rosemary, lavender and lemongrass. For emotional pain, ensure you use euphoric essential oils, to uplift and to numb some of the pain. Choose those oils very carefully. Florals and fruits tend to be most effective, although there are a few exceptions – benzoin is a wonderful aid against nightmares and for encouraging communication of feelings and thoughts in a peaceable way. Frankincense helps people to focus calmly and will generate a thoughtful response to any problem. Ginger is very useful when you feel that you would need a bomb lit under you to get you moving!

Anxiety

Feelings of anxiety can be debilitating. Anxiety makes it hard to relax, as there is a tendency to worry constantly. People tend to experience anxiety in different ways: sweating palms, racing heart, nervous diarrhoea, irritable bowel, skin breakouts, dry mouth, stuttering, being unable to remember what you were going to say – are all common responses.

The most effective essential oil for anxiety is neroli – and the expense of the oil is justified when you feel the results. Just inhale the fragrance to calm nerves within minutes. Other essential oils that are very effective for

anxiety include: mandarin, tangerine, orange, Roman chamomile, lavender, rose, benzoin, sandalwood, cedarwood, cypress.

Depression

The term 'depression' covers a continuum, ranging from a mild low (which might be brought on by pre-menstrual tension or emotional vulnerability and which can often be rescued by a cup of tea, some sympathy and a family-sized bar of chocolate) to a place where the person feels there is no hope. People at the far end of the continuum may be unable to see a way out of their situation, to think logically (or to think at all). They may have problems getting to sleep or spend a lot of time asleep, but not feel rested. Severe depression can take us to a point where we don't feel like dressing, taking basic care of ourselves, or doing anything – everything feels difficult. Depression in your friends or loved ones can be a very bewildering situation to face: there may be no logical explanation for why it would develop. When trying to help depression, ensure that you have some idea about how serious the depression is. One indicator is how long the person has experienced it. You must ask your friend if they are on medication: and if they are, you must ask them to consult their GP before proceeding. You may think it is appropriate to encourage the person to try other treatments (including counselling if they are open to this). All this information will help you make decisions about the choice of oils. Generally, euphoric oils are a must. You may find that even if the person is having trouble sleeping, strong sedatives like valerian will be un-suitable (and contraindicated if they are on medication for their depression). Use essential oils such as: rose, neroli, jasmine, orange, mandarin, tangerine, lemon, grapefruit, geranium, lavender, Roman chamomile, cypress, myrrh.

For mild depression:

- 🌿 mandarin 4 drops
- 🌿 sandalwood 2 drops
- 🌿 rose 2 drops

in 20 ml of carrier oil.

Insomnia

Very often, sleep is taken for granted until we aren't getting either enough of it or good quality of sleep. People develop the symptoms of insomnia for a large number of reasons (see the table below). Where it is long lasting, it is strongly recommended that you see your GP,

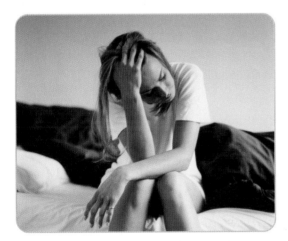

as insomnia can be linked to some more serious conditions. Useful essential oils for insomnia include: benzoin, clary sage, geranium, Roman chamomile, German chamomile, Atlas cedarwood, jasmine, lavender, mandarin, marjoram, neroli, orange, patchouli, petitgrain, rose, rosewood, sandalwood, spikenard, tangerine, valerian, vetiver, yarrow, ylang ylang. Generally, it is worth starting with lavender if you have trouble sleeping. If this doesn't work, move on to the stronger essential oils. Valerian is the last resort.

Anti-jet lag blend

This does not smell particularly pleasant, but if you have trouble sleeping on long-haul flights and know you need to have something to knock you out, make this up as a moisturiser for use everywhere you can reach, but especially on your face (and this is one time that I don't reduce the dosage for use on the face). Drink plenty of water on the flight and reap the benefits. A useful side-effect of this blend is that it is also very good at relieving aching muscles:

- 🌿 valerian 1 drop (or substitute with marjoram)
- 🌿 lavender 4 drops
- 🌿 German chamomile 3 drops

in 20 ml of moisturising lotion.

Common causes of insomnia	
Diet-related	Too much alcohol, caffeine, smoking, too much liquid drunk before bed (causing waking to urinate)
Pain-related	Arthritis, heartburn, heart diseases, osteoporosis, sinusitis, cancer, kidney disease, asthma
Nerve-related	Depression, Alzheimer's disease, Parkinson's disease, restless leg syndrome, dementia, sleep apnoea, incontinence
Environment-related	Stress, shift work, too many naps during the day

Headaches and migraines

Headaches arise for a number of reasons. Treating them can go beyond using lavender on a cool compress over your forehead. When your headache is self-inflicted as part of a hangover, then as well as drinking copious amounts of water, blending lavender and juniper or lemon together can be very helpful. Muscle tension headaches, where you can feel that the root cause of the problem is tension in your shoulders and neck which slowly creeps over your entire head, are very easily helped with aromatherapy – and the choice of essential oils is very wide. Choose muscle relaxants and analgesics by preference; for example, marjoram, sandalwood, lavender, Roman or German chamomile are all useful.

Migraines sometimes need a different approach. They arise for a number of reasons; sometimes as a result of stress, or possibly because of the presence of a trigger food such as chocolate, red wine or cheese. When they occur, the person will sometimes experience an 'aura' before it develops (this can be smelling an unusual smell, or a visual disturbance). If the migraine is in full swing, then use the strongest pain-killing essential oils that you have to hand, as long as they are also muscle relaxants and vasodilators (i.e. they dilate the blood vessels and reduce blood pressure). Lavender will help some people, but German chamomile, marjoram or (if you have it) valerian, are preferable. If you catch the migraine early enough, before it develops (as the aura arises), it can help to use an essential oil that is also a vasoconstrictor (i.e constricts blood vessels), as this can sometimes stop the migraine in its tracks. Cypress and peppermint are very helpful here – peppermint is very effective at reducing muscle spasms, too.

ME or chronic fatigue syndrome

Good results have been seen in cases of myalgic encephalomyelitis (ME), or chronic fatigue syndrome, by using food supplements (essential fatty acids – EFAs) and changes in diet and exercise levels as part of the treatment. As a person begins to recover from ME, aromatherapy massage can be regarded as 'light exercise', as you are working their muscles thoroughly as you treat them. Do not expect to be able to carry out a full body massage, as this may be exhausting for them. However, strong immune stimulants such as melissa, tea tree or lavender, when blended with essential oils that aid sleep (such as chamomile) and help depression or anxiety (neroli, for example), can be very effective in a blend. Dilute the blend to half the recommended dosage for an adult, as they may be very sensitive to the blend and the treatment. Try this blend:

- neroli 2 drops
- lemon 1 drop
- Roman chamomile 1 drop

in 20 ml of carrier oil.

Shingles

Although shingles might also appear as an immune disorder, it is listed here because it can be differentiated from normal chicken-pox in that it travels along the nerve pathways and emerges in specific areas as a very painful rash. Treat shingles with painkillers and strong immune stimulants – such as melissa, lemon, grapefruit, lavender, bergamot, cedarwood, Roman or German chomomile, or frankincense. Try this blend:

- bergamot (or melissa) 3 drops
- lavender 2 drops
- Roman chamomile 3 drops

in 20 ml of carrier oil.

Emotional swings

Emotional swings may be associated with fluctuating hormone levels, shock, high levels of stress, anxiety, manic depression and insomnia. If you are experiencing severe emotional swings you need to see a doctor to discuss how you are feeling. Where aromatherapy can help is if you use essential oils that are known to encourage a balanced emotional outlook. Geranium, frankincense, lemongrass, grapefruit, mandarin and neroli are all particularly good at this. Try them either as a massage blend or in the vaporiser to allow you to achieve a meditative state of mind when you are relaxing:

- geranium 2 drops
- neroli 2 drops
- orange 4 drops

in 20 ml of carrier oil.

Heartbreak

When we are on the road to emotional recovery we may reach a point where it feels as if the scales fall from our eyes and we can view the past with a different level of insight. Yet getting to that point can be very difficult. If you know someone in that position, they may appreciate one of the following blends. (Rose is strongly indicated for emotional recovery, but sometimes you need the stronger oils like ginger to give a bit of strength to go through with things.)

Finding the strength *not* to contact them:

- fennel 1 drop
- black pepper 4 drops
- rose 2 drops

in 20 ml of carrier oil.
Use this in the vaporiser day and night, too.

Convincing yourself that you are still attractive:

- jasmine 2 drops
- rose 1 drop
- patchouli 3 drops

in 20 ml of carrier oil.
Put jasmine in everything for a while – it blends very well with patchouli or vetiver to help re-establish sexual self-confidence.

Starting to notice the other fish in the sea

This blend helps when you first start to consider a new relationship after heartbreak. It will help you to stay emotionally present and to avoid comparing the new person with your previous partner.

- vetiver 2 drops
- jasmine 1 drop
- neroli 2 drops
- bergamot 3 drops

in 20 ml of carrier oil, or make up as a perfume.

Rage

We all have moments where we 'see red'. We may be seething for ages afterwards. Sometimes calming down is the hardest part. When that happens, we have a choice: a) throw the biggest tantrum we can; b) go somewhere and calm down until we can talk about whatever is bothering us in an effective (not tearful) way; or c) channel the energy into something productive. I've found the following blends useful.

After the tantrum – to clear the air:

- frankincense 3 drops
- juniper 5 drops
- orange 2 drops

(in water, to vaporise).

To calm down and plan an effective expression of what is bothering you:

- benzoin 2 drops
- palmarosa 4 drops
- rose 2 drops

in 20 ml carrier product (either in water, to vaporise, or in a moisturiser for use on your face and hands).

For lateral thinking – and channelling the energy elsewhere:

- palmarosa 3 drops
- frankincense (or basil) 3 drops
- grapefruit 4 drops

in water to vaporise.

Examination nightmares

I have recommended this blend to countless aromatherapy students who are about to take practical exams. The blend is very grounding and balancing. It helps to keep you focused, to keep nervous butterflies at bay and communicate effectively. As well as working as a massage blend, if you want to try applying each essential oil on its own to key areas pre-examination, try using the vetiver(neat) in your shoes, the neroli (1 drop in 5 ml of carrier oil) on your solar plexus and the sandalwood (1 drop in 5 ml of carrier oil) on your throat. It also works very well during driving tests.

- sandalwood 3 drops
- neroli 3 drops
- vetiver 2 drops

in 20 ml of carrier oil.

casestudy: Insomnia

Caroline came to class complaining about her inability to sleep. She said that the problems had started six weeks before, when she first came back from a long holiday. At first, she attributed the problem to jet lag, but when it didn't disappear after two weeks she became concerned. Further discussion made it clear that her insomnia was linked to a stressful job (which she was worried she was about to lose), anxieties to do with her children's schooling (they were awaiting news about which secondary school they would be allowed to attend). Caroline's insomnia had now reached the point that she was worrying about not being able to sleep. Volunteering herself as a 'group case study' she agreed to try any changes the class suggested for her.

The group agreed that Caroline needed to have an aromatherapy massage every three days for the next month. They felt this would be the optimum spacing between treatments. Because the essential oils would stay within Caroline's system for 72 hours, each treatment would be a 'top up' and would also allow them to monitor the effectiveness of the essential oils chosen. Between treatments, Caroline was to have a warm bath in the evenings before bed, using the same blend in the bath. She was also instructed to stop drinking any caffeinated drinks after 3 pm and to avoid alcohol altogether if possible (but if she did drink, not to exceed one unit).

As they would be taking it in turns to massage Caroline, the group agreed to a limited range of essential oils to work with and to keep in touch about the progress of the treatment.

Having considered a list of appropriate essential oils with sedating properties (see the table on page 14) in conjunction with the detailed information they gathered from questioning Caroline about her health and personal preferences, the group arrived at a shortlist of essential oils that they would use during her treatments. They intended to vary the blends each time, and that follow-up would involve Caroline commenting on any relative sleep improvements, as well as what she thought of the blend. Their shortlist included the following: benzoin, clary sage, geranium, chamomile – German and Roman varieties, jasmine, lavender, mandarin, marjoram, neroli, orange, patchouli, petitgrain, rose, rosewood, sandalwood, valerian, vetiver, ylang ylang.

The initial blend the group recommended was:
- clary sage 2 drops
- geranium 2 drops
- lavender 4 drops
in 20 ml of carrier oil.

These were chosen because the majority of the group had found lavender an effective sedative, because clary sage is structurally similar to a number of hormones, so it was felt that it might mimic the effects of melatonin (which is involved in maintaining the sleep–wake cycles) and geranium because Caroline liked the smell, it blended well with the other essential oils and was also sedating. Unfortunately, Caroline reported the next day that it hadn't worked at all, in fact she felt more depressed, tearful and exhausted.

This made the group more determined to find the right blend. Given Caroline's feedback, they decided that a much stronger sedating blend would be required. As a result, the next blend involved valerian, the strongest sedative in the collection and the plant substance from which Valium is derived. However, this had the opposite effect on Caroline. She said she was awake all night, rather than being able to doze, and felt very sad throughout. This was an unusual, although not an unheard of response   *cont.*

to valerian. (I have met clients in my own practice who are depressed and tend not to respond well to valerian, but there is little research information to justify or explain the response.) This pointed to the need to ensure that euphoric oils – those which lift the spirits – were a dominant part of the blend. The next blend produced a better result:

- jasmine 3 drops
- orange 3 drops
- petitgrain 2 drops

in 20 ml of carrier oil.

Following use of this blend, Caroline reported that her sleep had improved somewhat, that she felt more rested, but that she was still waking in the night and found that her mind was very restless. It was also taking a long time to fall asleep again. It was at this point that the group added cypress to their list of potential oils – cypress is indicated for overactive minds, even if it isn't always considered to be an effective sedative. Once cypress was introduced, Caroline reported that even if she did wake up in the night, she was able to fall back to sleep again without too much trouble. The blend that worked best for Caroline was:

- cypress 4 drops
- neroli 2 drops
- Roman chamomile 2 drops

in 20 ml of carrier oil.

Once Caroline's sleeping patterns improved, she reduced the number of treatments she received down to one every two weeks and she 'traded' treatments with another group member at this time.

Postnatal depression

Statistics suggest that some degree of postnatal depression is experienced by up to 20 per cent of women – and that there may be more who feel depressed but are able to hide it effectively from their GPs, health visitors, families and even from themselves. The strength of the symptoms varies from one woman to the next, as do the reasons that someone may develop it, but some of the common elements are:

- low self-esteem
- resentment/anger
- feelings of worthlessness
- tearfulness
- feeling numb
- insomnia
- loss of appetite
- loss of interest in other activities

ꙮ sexual disinterest

ꙮ occasionally, contemplation of suicide.

While aromatherapy and some other complementary therapies can help support a serious condition such as postnatal depression, it must be emphasised that these therapies cannot replace orthodox treatment. However, in conjunction with counselling, antidepressants (if prescribed) and nutritional support, you can help someone come through the depression and to re-establish their sense of equilibrium. Counselling is particularly recommended for this condition.

casestudy: Postnatal depression

Nadia came for course of five aromatherapy treatments on the recommendation of her counsellor, who had insisted that she needed to do something regularly that felt like a treat. The counsellor felt that aromatherapy would also help improve her sleep and reawaken her interest in her surroundings. Nadia had been diagnosed as depressed and was taking anti-depressants (she had just started to wean herself off the tablets after six months on them). What was most noticeable about her was that she looked (and said she felt) exhausted and that she had very little response to anything around her. She both felt and acted numb and did not volunteer much information. The challenge with Nadia was to help her sleep better, reawaken her lust for life and encouarge her to feel more positive about herself.

Choosing the essential oils to use with Nadia resulted in some interesting reactions. First, she couldn't stand either valerian or spikenard (both effective sedatives). She felt indifferent to most of the citrus essential oils (all considered to be euphorics) and initially didn't like the floral oils, which are particularly recommended to help balance hormonal fluctuations as well as easing depressive symptoms (She said that geranium, rose, jasmine and ylang ylang were all 'horrible'.)

The first blend used was:
ꙮ carrot seed 1 drop
ꙮ benzoin 3 drops
ꙮ neroli 4 drops
in 20 ml of carrier oil.

Carrot seed is an unusual oil and isn't always readily available. However, it is a very good sedative and has a particular affinity to the heart and to emotional distress.

Although Nadia responded well and said that she found the treatment enjoyable, it wasn't until the fourth treatment that we found a combination of essential oils that

cont.

93

were particularly effective at helping her to feel good, to sleep (thereby feeling more rested) and to have the energy to return to some of her previous activities. This blend involved another unusual oil – black spruce:

- black spruce 3 drops
- melissa 2 drops (this is expensive, lemon would be a cheaper substitute)
- sandalwood 3 drops

in 20 ml of carrier oil.

Black spruce is a relatively recent introduction to the list of essential oils available in Britain and has a very impressive track record where treating depressive states is concerned. Nadia loved it and was willing to use this blend in the bath between treatments, which she found helped to lift her spirits more effectively as she completed her course of counselling and found the balance between new motherhood and her own needs and desires.

Please note: If you suspect that someone may be contemplating taking their own life, discuss it with them, and, if appropriate, encourage them to seek immediate professional help.

FAQs – Aromatherapy for the mind and nervous system

I am really having trouble making decisions lately. Everything seems far more difficult than it used to be and I'm easily distracted. What can you suggest to help me focus and think clearly?

Try blending frankincense with a citrus oil such as lemon, tangerine, mandarin, grapefruit or orange. Put these in a vaporiser in an empty room – or at least one where there are no immediate distractions – and use that room for either meditating (if you are able to do this effectively) or just sitting down with your eyes closed. Take deep slow breaths and, when you are feeling calm, consider whatever the situation is objectively. You may find that a solution (or even a different way of looking at things) will emerge.

My memory at the moment is awful. I have exams coming up – what will help me learn more effectively?

This can vary. Generally, rosemary does help you to remember things (for example, it has been used effectively with people who are experiencing the first stages of senile dementia). However, it is not great to use last thing in the evening as it can interfere with your sleep. If late evening is the time you have allocated for learning, it might not be advisable to use it then. Try using another essential oil which will help you remain alert but calm – such as frankincense. You can also vary this by choosing a range of essential oils which you can associate with different topics that you are studying. If, for example, you have eight topics to cover, you could choose your eight favourite essential oils. Put the appropriate oil in the vaporiser with frankincense and you may find this helps. If you are consistent with your choice of essential oils each time you study, remembering the fragrance of the essential oil will remind you of the topic when it comes to the exam.

I would really like ten minutes' peace and quiet at the end of the day – what can I use to encourage my family to calm down and solve their own problems while I have a short break?

Try benzoin and cypress, possibly with geranium. Use these either in the vaporiser or put them on tissues and tuck it behind radiators (in the winter), or make a room fragrance (mix the essential oils with water and then mist the room) and spray that around the house before everyone arrives home.

My partner is under a great deal of stress right now and, when he comes home, he tends to be hypercritical. Can you suggest anything that will affect him quickly, calm him down and put him in a good mood?

If it is a quick response you want, you can either try a blend of clary sage, sandalwood, palmarosa and orange (2 drops of each in a vaporiser). Or, you may want to provide a more holistic approach – one which supports him properly. Later one evening, ask him to smell a selection of essential oils and say which he likes and make him feel calm, happy and stress-free. Use them in a vaporiser to fragrance the house before he gets home. More importantly, discuss what can be done to reduce his stress levels permanently, before it takes more of a toll on your personal relationship. (You may want to consult *Stress Management in Essence*, another book in this series.)

detoxification

'Detox' products are everywhere now, and the concept of using food, herbs, strange rituals and various complementary therapies in order to cleanse your body of impurities goes well beyond just the post-festive guilt trip when you become aware of how much you have ignored your body of late.

An effective regime designed to detox your system has to take into consideration a variety of organs and systems. These include:

- The lymphatic system – the secondary circulation system is responsible for picking up waste products from around the body and returning them to the blood so that they can eventually be removed via the kidneys as urine. It is also involved in the immune response.

- The kidneys – they may be working overtime to cleanse and filter your blood. If you haven't been drinking enough water, they may contain crystalline deposits that need to be removed from the body before they develop into kidney stones. Passing a kidney stone is very painful.

- The liver – responsible for virtually all chemical reactions relating to the detoxification of food, alcohol and all supplements (including prescribed and non-prescribed drugs), this organ is also associated with feelings of anger. Any effective detoxification regime will need to involve reducing the workload of the liver for a while. So you can expect to cut down on food high in additives, sugar, salt, and any substances that would also increase the burden on this organ.

- Reducing stress levels – when you are experiencing high levels of stress for an extended period of time, two adrenal hormones are released in large quantities to help your body cope with the problem. These hormones (cortisol – which raises blood sugar levels so you are prepared to fight or run away, and aldosterone – which alters how much water you retain, so that your body has some liquid to store toxins in until you are ready and able to release them) have a big impact on the body. In large amounts, cortisol makes skin problems worse, reduces the effectiveness of the digestive system and makes the reproductive system more prone to problems as well. The action of aldosterone encourages the body to retain water, so that when you are under stress, there is often an associated sense of bloating or water retention.

Aromatherapy can help to support the detoxification process in a number of ways. First, various oils with diuretic properties can help to reduce water retention, showing a particular affinity for the lymphatic system (and reducing the appearance of cellulite). Second, you can use specific essential oils to reduce cravings for the substances that are banned as you detox (for example, if you are craving chocolate, try blending geranium, benzoin and orange together). Third, the aromatherapy massage can be developed either to stimulate and energise the system (and reduce water retention), or to encourage you to relax and reduce stress levels.

Essential oils particularly useful to detoxify or reduce impurities are: rosemary, grapefruit, lemon, lime, orange, juniper, peppermint, lemongrass, fennel, angelica, bergamot, black pepper, rose, vetiver, sandalwood, cypress, eucalyptus, ginger.

Cellulite

For best effects, try dry skin brushing, followed by firm massage with the following:

- rosemary 2 drops
- grapefruit 2 drops
- juniper 4 drops

- (optional: angelica if you can get it – 1 drop)

in 20 ml of carrier oil.

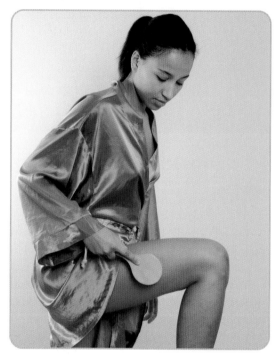

Skin brushing

Oedema and bloating

When oedema is particularly noticeable and problematic, it is important to consider how it developed, and why. Where bloating is pre-menstrual, you would be best to use essential oils that are closely linked to the reproductive system as well as being effective at detoxifying and reducing water retention. For example, try fennel, rose and orange (3 drops each of fennel and orange, 2 drops of rose). If you suspect bloating might be related to a particular food, then it is useful to speak to a nutritionist or to consider watching what you eat to see if you can spot the item that is responsible. Mild food intolerances sometimes cause bloating around the middle. Avoiding the substance in question can reduce bloating very quickly (the three most likely culprits are wheat, dairy products or eggs, but this is not always the case). If you know it is a food item that is causing the problem, then an anti-inflammatory essential oil – such as German chamomile, lavender or yarrow would be useful. Try lavender with juniper and geranium (equal amounts – 2 drops each in 20 ml).

casestudy: The New Year's resolution

Sonia had a particularly festive season one year and found herself feeling very hungover, lethargic and jaded on New Year's Day. She also felt that her cellulite had got markedly worse during the Christmas break and decided that she needed a concerted effort to return her body to a reasonable state of health as quickly and as painlessly as possible. As well as agreeing to give up alcohol for the next six weeks, she was attempting to quit smoking and wanted to improve her diet (although she suspected that this would prove to be unworkable in the face of all the other changes she wanted to make).

Treating Sonia for all the areas she expressed interest in required a great deal of commitment from her. As well as making the dietary changes she had highlighted, she was asked to do dry skin brushing and massage her own body (as much as she could reach) on a daily basis. She was also asked to drink at least 2.5 litres of water a day and to switch from tea and coffee to herbal teas. She booked in for one massage a week for six weeks. For the first session – a very vigorous treatment, designed to help motivate her as well as work on her cellulite – we used the following blend:

- rose 2 drops
- juniper 2 drops
- grapefruit 4 drops

in 20 ml of carrier oil.

Sonia was given the blend to use between treatments and was also persuaded to carry a bottle of lavender with her for the next two weeks, as it was likely that she could experience headaches and withdrawal symptoms from not having caffeine.

This blend worked well for Sonia, although she asked for a stronger blend to use between treatments that would really help to get her circulation going and to improve the appearance of her cellulite. We found that what worked best for her was to alternate (every other day) two very similar blends. The first one contained fennel, juniper and orange, the second contained rosemary, juniper and grapefruit.

cont.

99

We continued to use the rose blend in the treatment. At the end of six weeks, Sonia was very pleased as she noted an improvement in her energy levels, her sense of self-confidence, her muscle tone and her skin condition. Although she had finished the detox regime she had set herself, she was able to be more discerning about how much she took of the substances she had previously loved (her three chocolate-bars a day habit had diminished to one bar during the week she was premenstrual).

FAQs – About detoxing with aromatherapy

How long will it take to see a difference if I do the skin brushing and cellulite treatment?

This will depend on what other changes you are making at the same time. If this is the only thing you are doing, then you can expect your skin to be in much better condition within six to eight weeks. If you are changing your diet and exercise levels as well as doing the skin brushing and cellulite treatment daily (or twice daily), I would expect noticeable changes in four weeks or less.

Are there any side effects to doing an aromatherapy detox?

Yes, if you are doing it correctly, I would expect that you will be urinating more than usual (and the urine may be darker too). Don't forget to drink lots of water – at least two litres a day of plain water (or flavour it with lemon juice) – as this will reduce any unpleasant side effects, such as headaches.

Do I have to live on brown rice to detox effectively?

No, but it sounds as if the aspect of a detox that is bothering you the most is the changes to your diet. Speak to a professional nutritionist, as they may be able to help you find a way of detoxing that is effective and non-painful to you. You may also want to look at *Nutrition in Essence*, another book in this series.

I have cellulite and bloating on my belly. I don't have it anywhere else. What can I do to get rid of it?

Your muscles may be weak and need toning up. Abdominal massage will help, as well as exercise targeted at the area. For abdominal massage, try a blend of grapefruit (3 drops), black pepper (2 drops) and peppermint (3 drops) in 20 ml of carrier oil. It's also likely that you need to change some of the kinds of food you are eating (eat plenty of fresh vegetables), and look at how much and in what state of mind you eat. If you always eat when you are under stress you will be unable to digest your food properly, causing bloating. You may have a mild food intolerance which is causing your gut to become inflamed; you may want to see a nutritionist if you suspect this. If none of the above applies to you and you think you may be retaining fluid around your abdomen, you should check with your doctor.

muscular
aches and pains

Many people first approach aromatherapists because of muscular discomfort or pain. Most problems are in the back. Where this is the case, what people usually want is a lovely, long back massage – one which will reduce discomfort, help them relax and leave them smiling at the end of the treatment.

When you set out to treat muscular aches and pains, it is very important to get as much information as you can about exactly what is bothering the person you are about to treat. People sometimes hide their real reasons for having a treatment behind the 'safe excuse' of muscular tension, especially of the neck and shoulders. With muscular problems that may have developed as a result of physical overexertion, an effective treatment might a quite vigorous massage (all of which would be appropriate for an early morning treatment to leave the person feeling alert for the rest of the day). However, imagine a situation where someone says they have muscle tension, but

they haven't told you is that it is stress-related and that they had their first-ever migraine yesterday (and they are still in shock that this happened to them). Under these circumstances, a vigorous massage would not be appropriate; a far more gentle treatment would be indicated, even if they did want to remain alert for the rest of the day.

Essential oils for muscular aches and pains include: rosemary, peppermint, lemongrass, ginger, frankincense, valerian, black pepper, marjoram, vetiver, lavender, Roman chamomile, German chamomile, basil, cinnamon, clove.

Muscle strain

Overworked muscles are prone to strain, especially if they have not been properly warmed up. Try making a blend to work into muscles before exercise, to warm them up effectively, as well as using an analgesic blend to help recovery from strained muscles. This blend is dual purpose:

- ☙ black pepper 3 drops
- ☙ lavender 3 drops
- ☙ rosemary 2 drops

in 20 ml of carrier oil.

Sprains

When you sprain your ankle, you've damaged the ligaments that hold the bones together and in place over the joint. Ligaments have a relatively poor blood supply, which is why they take so long to heal. However, you can help the healing process somewhat by using analgesic essential oils such as lavender in a cold compress.

Arthritis

Arthritis is characterised by pain, stiffness and swelling of the joints. Osteoarthritis develops as a result of wear and tear on the joints. Usually, this is found in older people, although it can develop early if someone is overusing particular joints (athletes are prone to this), or if there has been a sudden weight gain. Although it can occur anywhere in the body, osteoarthritis tends to be found in weight-bearing joints or those that are subject

to overuse. Rheumatoid arthritis (or rheumatoid disease as it is sometimes called) is an autoimmune condition (where the body attacks itself) and causes pain over the whole body. In both cases, strong anti-inflammatory essential oils (such as yarrow, lavender, or chamomile) are indicated, as are painkillers (including rosemary, peppermint, black pepper, marjoram). However, with rheumatoid arthritis it is also useful to add essential oils that will regulate the immune system (for example, melissa, palmarosa, rosewood). In both cases, remind the person not to do any unusual activities after the treatment. Sometimes the reduction in pain can encourage them to make the most of their improved health and they may do too much, which might encourage a flare up of their condition.

For osteoarthritis:

- ☙ German chamomile 3 drops
- ☙ lavender 3 drops
- ☙ rosemary 2 drops

in 20 ml of carrier oil.

For rheumatoid arthritis:

- ☙ marjoram
- ☙ lemon
- ☙ Roman chamomile

in 20 ml of carrier oil.

Muscle tension and back pain

Always make sure you get to the bottom of what is causing the aches and pains people are experiencing. Massage will help muscle tension and back pain, especially if you use a warming blend which will soothe aching muscles and relax the individual. Try one of the following blends.

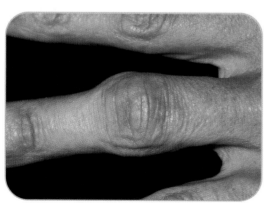
Arthritis in the hands

muscles, nerves and blood vessels from grinding against the underlying bone. Bursae tend to get inflamed if the joint is overused. The most common examples of bursitis are 'housemaid's knee' and 'tennis elbow'. Treatment with essential oils can involve cool compresses with anti-inflammatory essential oils, as well as a gentle massage with analgesic oils. Try this:

- lavender 4 drops
- yarrow 2 drops
- lemongrass 2 drops

in 20 ml of carrier oil.

Gout

Gout is a form of arthritis caused by a minor metabolic disorder. The pain, stiffness and swelling of joints associated with arthritis is limited to only a few joints (usually the ball of the foot, the ankle, the knee or the hip). Waste products of metabolism, namely uric acid and urate crystals, collect in the area and contribute to the pain. Although gout is more common in men than in women, in either case it is usually linked to a diet rich in red meat, salts, wine and other alcohols. Treating gout involves working not only with analgesic and anti-inflammatory essential oils, but also those which are very effective at improving the circulation and detoxing the system. Useful essential oils include juniper, fennel, angelica, grapefruit, lemon, lime, yarrow, German chamomile, lavender, black pepper and rosemary. Try this:

- juniper 4 drops
- rosemary 2 drops
- German chamomile 2 drops

in 20 ml of carrier oil.

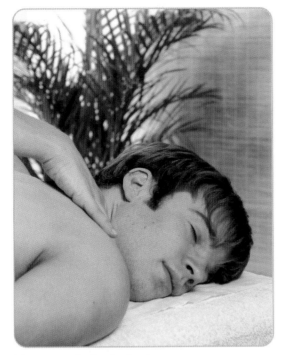

Massage to alleviate back pain

When you know that muscle tension or back pain is stress related:

- vetiver 3 drops
- lavender 2 drops
- neroli 3 drops

in 20 ml of carrier oil.

When the back pain is activity-related:

- German chamomile 2 drops
- black pepper 3 drops
- lavender 3 drops

in 20 ml of carrier oil.

Bursitis

Bursae are fluid-filled sacs or cavities that are found around most joints, where they protect

case study: The knee injury

A keen football player, Joe had been struggling with knee problems for a long time when he first came for treatment with aromatherapy. As well as practising a couple of times a week he had games every Saturday. He found he was coming to rely on over-the-counter painkillers that contained an anti-inflammatory (Ibuprofren) and was using them daily. While they did relieve the pain, Joe wasn't getting any better and he was missing more games and practice than he would like. The knee injury was also affecting his performance at work as he was getting more bad-tempered with the pain and because his major outlet for stress relief was reduced.

Until we carried out the consultation, Joe had been unaware of just how many painkillers he was taking, nor was he aware of how this could be contributing to other health problems he was starting to develop. He agreed to take two weeks off from football in order to allow himself to rest and recover effectively. In that time, he had three short aromatherapy treatments a week to work on reducing pain and inflammation as well as relieving stress. Joe's treatment involved two blends: a massage blend and one to use at home whenever the pain bothered him.

Massage blend:
- marjoram 2 drops
- German chamomile 3 drops
- lavender 3 drops

in 20 ml of carrier oil.

Home blend:
- German chamomile 7 drops
- lavender 7 drops
- eucalyptus 6 drops

in 20 ml of moisturising cream.

This second blend was very strong at 5 per cent in solution, but was only applied on and around the knees. Joe did not have sensitive skin.

Joe found the treatments very effective. He also found that the cream was a great help at reducing the pain and he was able to reduce the number of painkillers he took. We continued to use aromatherapy on him once a week after he returned to playing, but this was with mixed success. Joe eventually had to decide whether to face surgery or to give up playing as actively as he did. He chose the latter, and now coaches football (and is training as a sports massage therapist in his spare time).

FAQs – About muscular aches and pains

How would I know if someone isn't telling me the whole story about what is causing their pain?

Professional aromatherapists get around this issue by using a consultation questionnaire. This is a list of questions they ask before starting a treatment and covers everything from the client's contact details to a brief look at their medical history, their reasons for trying aromatherapy and the stressors in their life. It also shows if there are any contraindications to treatment. Sometimes, the questions may seem invasive. However, they are designed to show both the client and the therapist if there are any underlying patterns that might be contributing to whatever condition they are dealing with. Once they have completed the consultation, the therapist will usually ask the client to sign it. In signing it the client accepts that this is a true record of their health information as pertaining to the treatment. The therapist can only work with what they know, so it really is a good idea to be as truthful as possible.

If you are treating your friends and family it may be a good idea to design your own consultation questionnaire to make sure you have checked that it is safe to treat them. Going through the questionnaire a step at a time can also help you to pinpoint the areas where you suspect they aren't telling you the whole truth. Remember that they may well have reasons for not talking about something. Perhaps they feel shy or embarrassed. In cases like this, you may want to adjust your choice of essential oils to include ones which are suitable for anxiety, nervousness, or which are among the gentler oils (such as neroli and lavender), or which can move someone to feel confident enough to confide their worries (try benzoin or rose).

Confidentiality

If you are going to use a consultation sheet and work in this manner, then it is important to follow the same rules about confidentiality that a professional therapist follows. You should not share any of their personal details (spoken or written) with anyone else. Keep completed questionnaires under lock and key (where only you have access to the information). These rules are the basis of client confidentiality – a key tenet of professional behaviour among therapists.

Can you use essential oils to improve motivation and performance when you are working with serious athletes?

Yes, you can, although you will need to take close notes to uncover the reasons that are holding the athletes back from success. Most of the essential oils used for muscular aches and pains would be involved in a programme of improving athletic performance, as you would need to ensure that the athlete is in top physical condition just before (and after) an event. I've found ginger and black pepper in various combinations to be most useful at motivating those whose performance has been slightly 'sluggish'.

the respiratory system

Every time you have bought a pot of decongestant rub to help you recover from a cold, you have been engaging in aromatherapy. If you look at the ingredients, you will see that these rubs are chock-full of essential oils; usually a combination of rosemary, eucalyptus, wintergreen and camphor (both not commercially available as an essential oil) and occasionally, peppermint or lavender. Commercially produced decongestant rubs (and some other health products) can contain up to 40 per cent essential oils, which accounts in part for the powerful fragrance they emit. The blends suggested here, while much weaker at 2 per cent (or less), can be just as effective, not least because they will involve the gentler decongestant and expectorant essential oils, which will also help to clear your head and give you a good night's sleep.

Essential oils to help the respiratory system: rosemary, eucalyptus, tea tree, peppermint, sandalwood, cedarwood, rosewood, frankincense, lemon, orange, black pepper, cardamom, juniper, cypress, lavender.

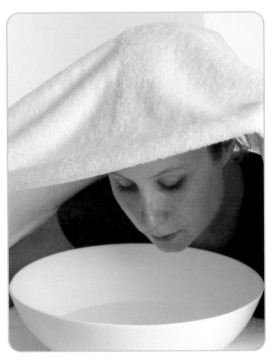

Inhalation will help clear your head

chapter thirteen

Sinusitis

Inflammation of the sinuses can lead to severe headaches as well as a stuffy nose and catarrh. Effective decongestants for sinusitis include: cardamom (the best), cypress, peppermint, ginger, lemon, orange, lime, bergamot and rosemary. Try this:

- cypress 1 drop
- cardamom 2 drops
- lemon 1 drop

in 20 ml of oil (for use on the face).

Sore throat

Nothing beats sandalwood for sore throats. Try using sandalwood on its own (or with lavender) – 4 drops in 20 ml of carrier oil – and applying it to the neck and behind the ears. You can reapply it as often as you like.

Bronchitis

Bronchitis usually develops after someone has had a common cold, virus or influenza. It is characterised by a deep and painful cough which is no longer as productive. Someone diagnosed as having chronic bronchitis will have had bronchitis for at least three months for two years running. In these cases, the usual decongestant blends do not help and you need something warming which will soothe the muscles and chest while gently clearing it. Frankincense is a must; cedarwood also helps, as do cardamom, orange, bergamot, sandalwood, rosewood, lavender and Roman chamomile. You can use these as a chest rub.

Coughs/colds

When you are feeling very run down, try vaporising this by your bedside at night. It will help to ease your chest, clear stuffy noses and get you a good night's sleep:

- marjoram 4 drops
- sandalwood 2 drops
- cedarwood 4 drops.

Tonsillitis

Tonsillitis inflames the lymphatic tissue at the back of the throat and can be very painful. This sensitive area is one of body's protective mechanisms designed to prevent invading viruses and bacteria from entering the body. When tonsillitis develops, it shows that the tonsils are working overtime to do the job they were designed to do. Other symptoms include swelling and in severe cases, the production of pus. Gargling with warm salt water can help to reduce the infection. (Some therapists add a drop of antiseptic essential oils to the salt water to increase the effectiveness of the treatment. However, this is not recommended unless the person can gargle without swallowing.) Essential oils such as lavender, sandalwood, lemon, German chamomile or tea tree are also useful as a concentrated blend to rub on the neck and as an inhalation.

For the throat:

- German chamomile 4 drops
- tea tree 4 drops
- lavender 4 drops

in 20 ml of carrier oil.

As an inhalation:

- sandalwood 1 drop
- tea tree 1 drop
- German chamomile 1 drop.

Catarrh

If someone is continually blowing their nose and coughing up sputum, try this blend for a facial oil (or vaporise the same oils at similar proportions). It will help to dry up the mucous and reduce the cough to more manageable levels:

- sandalwood 2 drops
- cypress 3 drops
- bergamot 3 drops

in 20 ml of facial oil.

FAQs – The respiratory system

I tend to get really bad bronchitis every winter. I've tried using rubs that are full of eucalyptus and rosemary, but they don't seem to help. What do you suggest?

Try using Atlas cedarwood (3 drops) and frankincense (1 drop); or marjoram (4 drops) in 20 ml of base oil. All three help to support the respiratory system and to ease painful coughing. You can use either of these blends as a chest rub.

I'm asthmatic. Which essential oils do you recommend to help me control my breathing before or during an asthma attack?

First, make sure you steer clear of eucalyptus, as this tends to interfere with the effectiveness of the most common asthma drugs prescribed today. Next, think about when you get the asthma attacks. Is it stress related? If so, I'd recommend neroli and frankincense as a blend to rub onto your chest. Is it related to food or household products? In these cases you may want to avoid the triggers and look at vaporising essential oils such as lemon or juniper to clear the environment. When you do experience an attack, vaporising frankincense, cedarwood and marjoram together can work wonders.

Can you suggest anything that would help me while I try to give up smoking?

Vetiver is very useful if you are trying to overcome cravings. If you find you are irritable, try neroli, tangerine, mandarin or grapefruit. Use a vaporiser regularly with essential oils that can encourage a calm atmosphere (and help you breathe more deeply), such as sandalwood or frankincense.

the immune system

The body's immune defences are governed by the lymphatic system, which, as well as making white blood cells and antibodies to all manner of diseases and pathogens (disease-causing organisms), also functions as a secondary circulation system. It is responsible for picking up any waste products from the body cells and tissues and returning them to the blood, where they can be sent to the kidneys for filtering and removal from the body.

Sometimes, the actions of the immune system can be irritating to the body – one of the first things it does when there is an invading organism is to develop an inflammation in the surrounding tissues. If it is a cold virus, for instance, you might see inflammation of the nasal passages, the mucus membranes and the sinuses. Sinus headaches, runny noses, aching joints (or lymph nodes) are the first signs that you are coming down with something.

Some conditions, such as HIV/Aids or certain types of cancer, can make catching a cold a life-threatening prospect. In these cases, the person's immune system can be so inadequate that they are unable to fight the cold. A 'simple' cold could escalate into bronchitis or pneumonia and may even be life-threatening.

Feeling feverish

Sometimes it is necessary to sweat out a fever. Try this blend in the bath, then wrap up warm and go to bed. It will make you sweat things out, but you will feel significantly better in the morning:

- black pepper 2 drops
- tea tree 3 drops
- lemon 1 drop

in a full bath.

Inflammation

Inflammation arises from many causes – including sprained ankles, strained muscles, acne and ingrown toenails. Despite the fact that the inflammation is sometimes needed (for example, it will help to keep a broken bone in place in order to allow it to heal properly), there are occasions where it is necessary to reduce the inflammation: perhaps the body is over-reacting (as is the case with hay fever), or there is pain to be relieved. Both German chamomile and yarrow are the best at reducing inflammation. The characteristic blue colour of these essential oils arises because they both contain chamazulene, a chemical which is a powerful anti-inflammatory agent. Juniper, lavender and marjoram are also useful.

Allergies

An allergic reaction can take several forms – from the most severe anaphylactic shock, which will require immediate medical attention – to milder examples, such as hay fever. In all cases, the body is over-reacting to the presence of an allergen. As a result, there is always some form of inflammation. Allergic reactions can include skin reactions such as hives, increased mucous production, itchy eyes, sneezing, or, in the case of food allergies, bloating, a change in the bowel habits and occasionally associated mood swings. Allergies respond well to blends that include essential oils like lavender, German or Roman chamomile, yarrow, cedarwood, cypress, tea tree, rosewood. For food allergies, try peppermint or juniper.

Hay fever

Hay fever is a hypersensitive reaction to something in the environment, usually pollen. In this case your immune system is working overtime. Treating hay fever tends to involve using anti-inflammatory essential oils, as well as those which dry up mucus. Try this:

- juniper 2 drops
- cypress 2 drops
- lavender 4 drops

in 20 ml of carrier oil.

Candida

Candida albicans is a yeast which colonises our digestive tracts within days of birth. It can become a problem if it takes over and does not allow space for the other digestive bacteria to grow. People tend to notice problems with candida infections when they are run down, or following bacterial or viral infections (especially if they have been given antibiotics). The antibiotics will kill off most bacterial life within the digestive tract. However, candida is like the dandelion plant: very difficult to remove. Symptoms of a candida overgrowth include bloating; digestive discomfort; oral, vaginal, or penile thrush; and athlete's foot. Treating systemic candida (where it involves the digestive tract) involves far more than aromatherapy can achieve alone: dietary support will be required. However, abdominal massage can help, especially if you use essential oils that are strongly recommended for their ability to deal with fungal infections: Try this blend:

🕉 tea tree 4 drops

🕉 bergamot 2 drops

🕉 lemongrass (or peppermint) 2 drops

in 20 ml of carrier oil.

Oral thrush responds well to mouth washes – use a drop of tea tree swirled within a large glass of water (be careful not to swallow). Vaginal or penile thrush are best dealt with using tea tree or lavender in a warm bath. Mild cases of vaginal thrush can respond well to one drop of lavender on a tampon, which is then inserted for four hours (allow a four-hour break after this). Please note that if your thrush is severe, this is not recommended. The mucous membranes lining the walls of the vagina are very sensitive and even lavender could be an irritant if the thrush is severe and widespread.

FAQs – Supporting the immune system

I tend to get every bug going around each winter. What essential oils are useful for me?

You need a blend of essential oils that will really boost your immune system. Try black pepper, melissa, lemon, tea tree, grapefruit, eucalyptus or cedarwood. You could try putting a couple of drops on a tissue and keeping it in your clothes so that the smell stays with you throughout the day.

I tend to get terrible vaginal thrush. What will work for this?

Try using lavender and tea tree in equal amounts (2 drops each) in a warm bath. You might also want to think about how you usually care for this area. A lot of soap or bubble bath can make thrush worse (so just use clear water). If you don't already wear it, cotton underwear is preferable to synthetic fibres.

I get cystitis all the time. I'm afraid that if I'm not careful it may escalate into a kidney infection. Can you recommend anything?

A great treatment for cystitis involves a warm bath with geranium, sandalwood and juniper (2 drops of each). However, don't forget to use other remedies as well: drink lots of water (or cranberry juice), and keep the area clean.

the endocrine system

The endocrine system is responsible for the manufacture of hormones – chemical messengers that travel around the body via the blood, causing changes in their target organs. Hormones are responsible for most of the changes that occur in the body as a result of growth, development and reproduction – and much more. As you saw in Chapter 10, the nervous system responds to immediate changes in the body or its environment: the endocrine system fine-tunes these changes.

Essential oils can be very effective at supporting some endocrine disorders. Some oils are very similar in structure to hormones. (This is particularly true of the endocrine hormones that govern the reproductive system: clary sage, fennel, jasmine and rose are extremely useful at dealing with disorders of this nature.)

SAD

Seasonal affective disorder (SAD) syndrome affects people as the seasons change and winter draws in. It is sometimes linked to changes in the amount of melatonin produced by the pineal gland. The symptoms, which can vary widely, include: insomnia, anxiety, tearfulness, restlessness and depression. Try using essential oils that the person associates with sunshine or summer gardens. Warming and uplifting oils such as Roman chamomile, ginger, black pepper, orange, grapefruit, jasmine, geranium or lemongrass are all helpful.

Thyroid problems

Thyroid problems, especially hypothyroidism (where the body isn't producing enough thyroid hormones), are sometimes difficult to recognise. With hypothyroidism, for example, you might experience lack of concentration, sluggish memory, a slow but steady weight gain, a desire to sleep for long periods (without feeling rested) and changes in the quality of your skin. By contrast, the

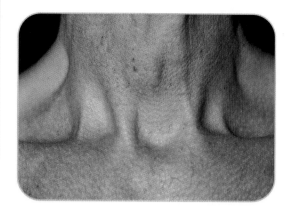
Swollen thyroid glands

opposite is true when you have hyper-thyroidism – your heart might race, you will lose weight, sweat more and feel anxious. If you suspect you may have problems with your thyroid, it is important to speak to your GP and get the appropriate blood tests if they believe that you may have a problem. In the meantime, you can use essential oils to improve your concentration (rosemary, eucalyptus, lemon – try these in the vaporiser), Exercise will help to improve the quality of your sleep and help to keep your weight steady (try juniper and grapefruit to aid any detox efforts here). For hyper-thyroidism, nothing beats ylang ylang for its ability to reduce heart palpitations and a racing pulse. Mix it with cypress if you know you are sweating a lot, and choose other essential oils designed to calm and soothe the whole system. Lavender will be very useful.

The adrenal glands

The adrenal hormones are most closely associated with their involvement in the stress response, although these tiny glands make a great many other hormones. Adrenalin and noradrenalin are responsible for our immediate response to perceived danger (whether physical, mental or emotional). Aldosterone helps to adjust the concentration of certain minerals in the body. When we are under a great deal of stress, aldosterone is involved in helping the body retain additional water to store the toxic by-products of our altered metabolism as we work under 'emergency' conditions. Cortisol adjusts blood sugar levels to cope with long-term stress.

Dealing with over-active adrenal glands using aromatherapy is best done using a blend of euphoric and uplifting essential oils in combination with deeply sedating oils that are also muscle relaxants. Try any of the citrus oils or jasmine, rose, neroli and muscle relaxants such as marjoram, German or Roman chamomile. This blend really works:

- clary sage 2 drops
- marjoram 2 drops
- Roman chamomile 2 drops
- orange 2 drops

in 20 ml of carrier oil.

Also, try having the orange essential oil in the vaporiser while you are working.

Try this

You can get an idea of how your current stress level is affecting your body by borrowing a tip from reflexology.

Try hooking into (pressing hard with the thumbs and moving with a caterpillar-like motion), rotating on the reflex points relating to the adrenals on either your hands or your feet. Most people, no matter how relaxed they believe themselves to be, experience some pain at this point – usually a dull, nagging pain. If the pain is intense, then it is time to start dealing with what stress is doing to your body, either through regular treatments and/or by approaching the stressors head on.

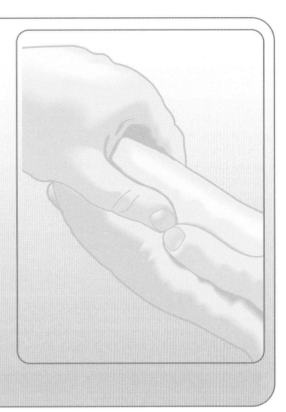

The adrenal reflex points

casestudy: Polycystic Ovarian Syndrome (PCOS)

Monica was diagnosed with PCOS when her GP did some blood tests and sent her for a scan to find out why she appeared unable to conceive. The list of symptoms she was told someone with PCOS could develop was certainly off-putting: lack of periods, infertility, (occasionally) early menopause, obesity and increased growth of hair (usually 'male pattern hair growth', which women notice on their faces, chest and groin area).

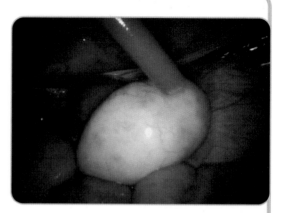

While the diagnosis did mean that Monica could go on the waiting list for assisted fertility, the waiting period was so long that she also decided to try aromatherapy to see if it could improve her chances of conceiving naturally.

PCOS is sometimes termed an insulin-resistant disorder. In the context of aromatherapy, this means two things: first, that the woman is producing too much insulin (the hormone involved in regulating the amount of sugar in our blood) and that this is affecting the balance of all the other hormones in her body; and second, that although alternative therapies can help to reduce stress (increased levels of stress cause a complex reaction in our bodies which results in higher levels of sugar in the blood) and adjust hormonal balance, they won't work in PCOS unless the diet is also addressed. In Monica's case, this meant she would need to make a huge reduction in the amount of carbohydrates she ate. As she was vegetarian and had a very sweet tooth, this was going to be difficult!

Treating Monica with aromatherapy involved making a plan to give her regular aromatherapy massages for a three-month period (hormonal changes are often relatively slow to come about so you need to see the person for a longer time to check the treatment is working properly), as well as a range of aromatherapy products she could use between treatments. As the cost of treatment was an issue, we decided that Monica would have one treatment every 10 days to 2 weeks, starting the first treatment in the week after her period stopped. She would also have two products to use at home between treatments – a bubble bath and a body moisturiser, both of which were to be used daily (with the body moisturiser used predominantly on her abdomen). Monica felt that she wasn't ready to see a nutritionist just yet, but after researching PCOS on the internet, she decided to eat a protein meal at breakfast, increase her intake of water and cut sweets, cakes, biscuits and alcohol down to an absolute minimum, allowing herself one treat per week.

Each massage treatment involved a slightly different range of essential oils, to take account of how Monica was feeling, where she was in her menstrual cycle and how she had responded since the last treatment. I gave Monica a new bubble bath and moisturiser at each treatment (for use until the next treatment). Monica responded best to a small number of oils: rose (she loved this, and it is a very effective menstrual regulator and improves fertility); clary sage and fennel (both are structurally similar to oestrogen and were great in separate blends, though they don't smell good together); damiana (a fantastic essential oil to treat reproductive problems, but is now almost impossible to get hold of); grapefruit and vetiver (both are invaluable aids to cleanse the body of toxins and vetiver also helps reduce cravings if you are trying to control an addiction, as well as having certain aphrodisiac qualities).

Within three months, Monica noticed a number of changes. For the first two weeks, she found the changes to her diet very difficult. After that, she found that she wasn't craving sugar as much. She also noticed that having protein at breakfast helped her to feel less hungry later in the day and she stopped wanting a sweet snack in the mornings. While some weight did come off, it wasn't a huge amount. However, Monica was pleased because it all came off her waist and abdomen, something she puts down to the change in diet coupled with the daily abdominal massage. She loved the aromatherapy massage and using the products and noticed that she felt far calmer and was able to sleep better as a result. Her periods did become more regular, and she had three periods in three months (whereas before she would have a period every six to eight weeks). At the end of the fourth month, she became pregnant naturally.

One of the blends Monica particularly liked (and which we used both as a bubble bath and as a massage blend was:
- rose otto 3 drops
- vetiver 3 drops
- fennel 2 drops

in 20 ml carrier oil, or 20 ml bubble bath solution.

FAQs – About aromatherapy and the endocrine system

I have diabetes, can you use essential oils to improve this?

There is nothing, as yet, to show how essential oils could be used to take the place of the insulin that I assume you are taking, or that would encourage your pancreas to resume making the amounts of insulin that you need. However, aromatherapy can help with some of the symptoms you may be experiencing. Massage can help to lower blood sugar levels. If your peripheral circulation (to your hands and feet) is a problem, rosemary or black pepper can improve it.

What can aromatherapy do to reduce the amount of cortisol in my body? I have read that this hormone is responsible for stress.

Cortisol is an adrenal hormone that helps to turn proteins and fats into sugar and to keep the blood sugar levels elevated so that you have the energy you need to cope with whatever stressors you face. Cortisol is present in large amounts if you are under a great deal of stress and have been for a long time. It is necessary to help you cope with stress, but prolonged exposure to high levels of it is what brings on stress-related disorders. Reducing cortisol levels and the effects of those stress-related disorders

only happens when you make the lifestyle changes necessary – like dealing with what is causing the stress in the first place.

When cortisol levels are high, changes in the body occur, particularly to the skin, reproductive system and digestive system. Stress-related conditions such as acne, eczema, infertility, irregular periods or irritable bowel syndrome (IBS) are just some of the things that can develop. You can use aromatherapy to treat stress and for whichever conditions have developed as a result of the stress. (Check the index – all of the conditions mentioned here are discussed elsewhere in the book.) However, the only way to significantly reduce cortisol levels is to deal with the situations that are causing stress.

Can you use aromatherapy to help my daughter grow faster? She is one of the smallest people in her class.

No. Massage will relax her, help improve blood supply to the muscles and bones of her body and facilitate the passage of growth hormone around her system. However, give her a chance to grow naturally. (NB: taking synthetic growth hormone has a number of side effects and should only be considered as a last, and desperate, resort.)

the reproductive system

When you consider that flowers are the reproductive organs of a plant, then it is not hard to see the link between some of the most glorious essential oils that we have available to us and their effectiveness in supporting the health and well-being of the reproductive system. Our reproductive health is something that forms a central part of our lives from the moment that puberty arrives. Teenagers are faced with the clash of examination pressures and hormonal rushes as oestrogen (in girls) and testosterone (in boys) suddenly flood their systems. Body parts they previously ignored start to grow in unexpected ways; the adjustment process takes time and patience (not least in their parents). As we get older, the question of fertility becomes a serious issue: to avoid becoming pregnant when you don't want to be; and to get pregnant quickly and easily when you decide that this is what you want. When these things don't work out according to plan, the emotional fall-out can be hard.

Menarche

Menarche is the term used to describe the onset of puberty in girls. Sometimes, the sudden changes in her body can be a real shock for a young woman. Not all can easily accept these changes. This is a time when parents or guardians are advised to keep a close eye on their charges: young women who aren't yet comfortable with having an adult body and the responsibilities that go with it occasionally develop eating disorders such as anorexia. (But note that eating disorders can arise as a reaction to other forms of distress.) Anorexia can result in periods stopping altogether until normal weight returns.

Accepting the changes

Helping a young woman adjust to her changing body can take time. Aromatherapy is very effective in supporting this, but you do need to adjust the choice of essential oils slowly over a period of time. Start with the fruit oils and work towards the florals (ending with rose or jasmine, the most overtly feminine essential oils in the list given below) as the young woman grows more comfortable with her body. You may want to try introducing the oils in the following order (try a different blend each week):

grapefruit
↓
bergamot
↓
orange
↓
tangerine
↓
neroli
↓
geranium
↓
ylang ylang
↓
rose
↓
jasmine

Try using your choice of the above essential oils in the following blend. The blend will help her feel emotionally grounded, less anxious and will also aid sleep.

- ꙮ an essential oil of your choice from the list above: 3 drops
- ꙮ lavender: 3 drops
- ꙮ frankincense: 2 drops

in 20 ml of carrier oil.

Regulating periods

It sometimes takes several years for the menstrual cycle to regulate following menarche, especially if the young woman is underweight, very physically active or experiencing exam stress (or similar). Some of the most effective emmenagogues (essential oils which bring on menstruation) and menstrual regulators are geranium, rose, jasmine, clary sage and fennel. Try this blend:

- ꙮ geranium 2 drops
- ꙮ sandalwood 4 drops
- ꙮ clary sage 2 drops

in 20 ml of carrier oil.

Hormonal tantrums

Whether a teenager is male or female, burgeoning hormones can lead to a lot of stress, tension and aggression within any household. The most effective essential oil for reducing tension of this kind (or allowing it to be dispersed in a relatively pain-free manner) is benzoin. Use it in a vaporiser, especially if there is a particular room where any fights tend to occur. You can also blend it effectively with frankincense (encourages a calm, meditative state) and palmarosa (diffuses anger). Try this blend:

- ꙮ benzoin 3 drops
- ꙮ frankincense 2 drops
- ꙮ palmarosa 3 drops

in 20 ml of carrier oil (or use the same ratio of drops in water to vaporise).

Infertility

Infertility, or sub-fertility, as it is sometimes called, is an increasingly common issue.

Research in this area has linked sub-fertility to a number of issues.

Age

More people are waiting to start a family until after they have reached certain goals they set for themselves. When you consider that women are at their most fertile when they first start to menstruate as teenagers, and that this fertility drops off with age, it does not seem so surprising that it can take some time for a couple in their thirties to conceive naturally.

Diet

A diet high in vegetables and fruit tends to include more of the trace vitamins and minerals that support fertility. Improvements to diet in order to aid fertility usually involve reducing caffeine, sugar, nicotine and gluten (a protein found in variable proportions in many cereals, for example wheat and rye) and increasing water and fruit intake.

Recreational drugs

Over-consumption of alcohol reduces fertility in both men and women (more so in women). Cannabis reduces sperm motility in men and prevents sperm from penetrating the capsule surrounding the egg.

Percentage of body fat

People at both ends of the spectrum (those who are clinically obese and those who are underweight and have little or no body fat) tend to be less fertile.

Stress

This is the biggest factor affecting fertility today. High stress levels reduce sexual drive as well as alter menstrual cycles and affect sperm production.

Aiding fertility in women

I have found rose and vetiver, when used together (even at relatively low dilutions) to be the most effective blend for women who are trying to conceive. In fact, it has been so successful that I have rarely had to use any other blend on clients in this position. As well as using this blend as part of a massage, self-massage of the abdominal area (or back massage if you have a willing partner) is also extremely useful, as is putting the blend in a bath. Alternative choices include jasmine, neroli, patchouli, or fennel, depending on your personal preferences. Try this blend:

- rose 3 drops
- vetiver 3 drops

in 20 ml carrier oil.

Aiding fertility in men

The process of trying to get pregnant may appear to be centred on the woman, but the effects of the process on the male partner should not be neglected. This can be a very trying time for them, especially if they are under stress in other areas of their lives, or if conception does not occur as quickly as desired. The following blend is very supportive, not only to the male reproductive system but also to the emotions and psyche (and it is loaded with aphrodisiac oils):

- clary sage 2 drops
- sandalwood 4 drops
- black pepper 2 drops

in 20 ml carrier oil.

Aphrodisiacs

There are an extraordinary number of essential oils that are known to be aphrodisiacs, not all

123

of which will work for everyone. Aroma-therapy is considered to be a holistic treatment – which means that the responses of the individual are paramount in how the treatment develops. If you are looking for an essential oil (or selection) which will help you relax and feel sexually receptive, your best bet is to do a smell test (see page 28) on a range of essential oils to see which ones encourage these feelings for you. (For example, one group of students I know who carried out this exercise several years ago, decided that the blend that worked best along these lines for all of them was black pepper, tea tree and lemon. This surprised me, as I would have chosen that blend to treat the symptoms of the common cold!) Each of the blends suggested here has at least one essential oil in it that is known for its aphrodisiac qualities:

- black pepper 3 drops
- ylang ylang 3 drops
- orange 2 drops

in 20 ml carrier oil.

- vetiver 2 drops
- jasmine 2 drops
- melissa (or lemon) 4 drops

in 20 ml carrier oil.

- patchouli 3 drops
- rose 3 drops
- bergamot 2 drops

in 20 ml carrier oil.

Supporting pregnancy and labour

As you will remember from Chapter 3, pregnancy may be a contraindication to treatment. You should proceed with caution, according to the personal circumstances of the individual. Generally, if someone has no history of unstable pregnancies or miscarriages and they are in good health, they can benefit from aromatherapy during pregnancy. However, it is wise to avoid using essential oils on the skin during the first trimester. After you enter the second trimester (at four months), it is possible to use essential oils (assuming the pregnancy is progressing normally), but they must be used at 1 per cent (or less) in solution – half the recommended dilution for a healthy adult.

> The essential oils that are safe for use in pregnancy are: cardamom, chamomile (Roman and German), clary sage, coriander seed, geranium, ginger, lavender, neroli, palmarosa, patchouli, petitgrain, rose, rosewood, sandalwood.
>
> Avoid these otherwise 'safe' oils if the person has a history of miscarriage: chamomile, clary sage, cypress, jasmine, juniper, lavender, marjoram, nutmeg, peppermint, rose, rosemary.

Morning sickness

'Morning sickness' can happen all day and, in particularly unlucky cases, goes well beyond the first trimester. Ginger or peppermint oil are particularly effective at dealing with nausea. The choice of which to use will vary with the person's taste. Ginger or peppermint tea is also helpful at this time.

Adapting to new circumstances

Whether the pregnancy is planned or otherwise, the immediate sense of impending change in one's life may require neroli to calm the butterflies.

Insomnia

Insomnia during the first trimester is often linked to an increased need to urinate at night. This does calm down during the second trimester (but comes back in the third). Try putting a drop of lavender and a drop of geranium or sandalwood on a tissue and placing it in your pillow case.

Lethargy

Lethargy and exhaustion are common in the first trimester, especially at the very beginning, before your blood supply alters to take into account the needs of the foetus. This is also nature's way of getting you to slow down. Try a drop of frankincense and black pepper on a tissue.

Stretch marks

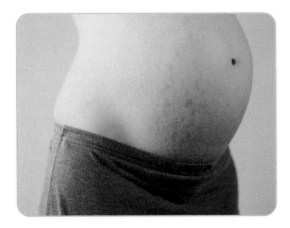

Simply oiling the skin with a carrier oil can help to reduce the appearance of stretch marks

during pregnancy and make sure that they disappear afterwards. The most effective carrier oil for this purpose is calendula oil. Use the carrier oil on its own if the skin is very sensitive or tends to be dry and already stretched uncomfortably during the first trimester. In the second trimester you can add essential oils to enhance the effects of the treatment. This blend can also be useful at reducing the appearance of the stretch marks even years after giving birth. Try this:

- frankincense 4 drops
- lavender 3 drops
- neroli 3 drops

in 60 ml carrier oil.

Or this:

- lavender 2 drops
- sandalwood 1 drop
- mandarin 1 drop

in 20 ml of carrier oil.

The second trimester

The second trimester is the time at which women notice the most changes to their bodies (especially first-time mothers). With any luck, the morning sickness will have stopped. After 20 weeks, prospective mums start to look 'properly' pregnant. They may notice some strange aches and pains – most of which can be helped with regular massage – this may be the only time in your life that you can get your partner to give you regular massage without complaining – take advantage of the situation! Gentle exercise, especially yoga for pregnancy, also helps.

Pubic discomfort

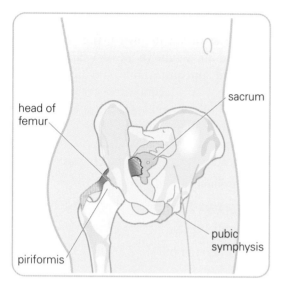

Location of pubic discomfort

Constipation

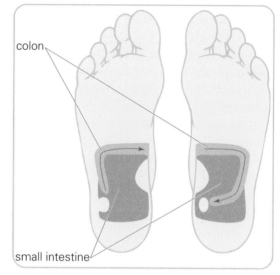

Reflex points for colon and small intestine, hooking-movements on arrows as shown

Some women experience discomfort in the pubic symphysis (the point at which the pubic bones join, right above the labial area of the vagina). This is usually as a result of the presence of the hormone relaxin, which is released at this point in the pregnancy. Relaxin causes the ligaments to stretch around key joints in the body – notably the hips. This helps to widen the hip area so that there is more space for the baby to travel down the birth canal during labour. The pain is a dull ache and may last for several days (and may also be experienced in the lower back around the sacrum or in the side of the buttocks directly over the heads of the femurs (the long bones in the thighs). This needs a blend that includes essential oils that are muscle relaxants, analgesics and anti-inflammatories. Try this:

- German chamomile 3 drops
- lavender 2 drops
- marjoram 3 drops

in 40 ml of carrier oil.

Constipation is a common problem as a pregnancy develops. The increased size of the uterus forces the intestines into a smaller space within the abdominal cavity, making it harder for the woman to completely (and easily) empty her bowels. Increasing water intake helps immeasurably (as does an increase in fibre in the diet). Massaging the abdomen and the base of the feet with a combination of geranium, grapefruit and Roman chamomile also helps to ease this condition. (If you massage the feet as shown in the diagram, you will also stimulate the reflexology points relating to the digestive system. For further advice about using reflexology, see *Hands on Reflexology*, by Andrew James). Try this:

- geranium 2 drops
- grapefruit 3 drops
- Roman chamomile 3 drops

in 40 ml of carrier oil.

Third trimester

Early on in the last trimester, women often report feeling at their best during the pregnancy. They tend to be sleeping well – at least until they get too heavy to rest comfortably, which happens near the end of the pregnancy. Their libido has often returned, as has their appetite.

High blood pressure

Many women experience raised blood pressure during their pregnancy. It is normal for the blood pressure to rise a little, but it is dangerous to the mother and the baby if it rises too much. It can be an indication of more severe conditions, such as pre-eclampsia. If you have been getting headaches, and you know your blood pressure is higher than it was (or should be), you need to discuss it with your midwife or doctor urgently. If you know your blood pressure is raised or if there is a family tendency to raised blood pressure during pregnancy, you may find it useful to use either ylang ylang or neroli in the bath regularly. Both essential oils are very effective at reducing blood pressure. You only need to use one or two drops in a full bath of water to get the benefits of this treatment.

Swollen ankles/wrists

Many women in the latter stages of pregnancy experience some oedema, especially in the hands and feet. This can be related to the weather, sudden weight changes, to changes in blood pressure or as a result of the level of activity in their lives (less active women or those in sedentary jobs tend to suffer more from oedema). Although peppermint or rosemary are very effective at reducing swelling, both essential oils raise blood pressure and should be avoided if you are experiencing raised blood pressure. They are also rather harsh on the skin if you have sensitive skin. The following blend is effective and mild for use at this time:

- grapefruit 2 drops
- juniper 1 drop
- geranium 1 drop

in 20 ml of carrier oil.

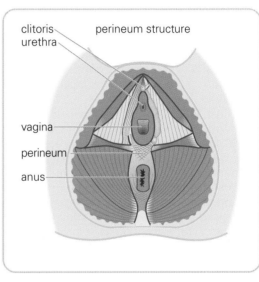

The perineum

Perineal massage

Many midwives and champions of natural birthing methods swear by the effectiveness of perineal massage. The purpose of the treatment is to soften and prepare the perineal region in anticipation of the birth. Massaging this area will increase blood circulation to the area, encourage the tissue to grow and be more elastic, making it more likely that the mother can deliver the baby without needing an episiotomy (where the doctor or midwife cuts the perineum in order to increase the area through which the baby will emerge). If you are keen to try this treatment yourself, you will need to massage the whole of the perineum up to and including the edge of the anus. Because this is a membranous surface,

it is more porous to essential oils, which is why the following blend is so dilute:

✄ lavender 1 drop

in 100 ml carrier oil (calendula oil is a good choice).

FAQs — About the reproductive system

My son has just reached puberty and is most distressed by the effects it is having on his skin. He seems to have severe acne now, regardless of what he eats. What can I do to help?

There is quite a bit you can do to help hormone-related skin conditions (see page 68 for further information). In your son's case, the obvious solutions involve encouraging him to drink more water to flush out any toxins that may be present and to reduce his intake of sugary or salty snacks and sweet drinks. You can also make him some skin care products (see pages 71–72) which include essential oils that both cleanse the skin and balance hormones (and, naturally, smell suitably masculine). If he's prepared to try a proper cleansing routine, then make a cleanser, toner and moisturiser for him. However, if he only wants to use one product, then make a shower gel (which he can use all over, including on his face), and one 'cream' to use in the daytime. Try blending sandalwood, palmarosa and bergamot or

juniper (2 drops each in 20 ml of carrier oil – ideally jojoba, but see Chapter 7 for other ideas). Sandalwood, bergamot and juniper are all antiseptic, helping to kill any bacteria on the skin as well as balancing the skin's production of sebum. Palmarosa will calm and soothe reddened areas as well as reducing infection.

My partner has been giving me aromatherapy massages throughout my pregnancy, which has been great. However, I'm now overdue. Can aromatherapy start labour?

Yes, it can. In my own practice I have created blends that can bring on labour within a day (although, in complete honesty, the blend in question didn't work for me when it was my turn to give birth!) However this is a situation that requires a lot of support, advice and guidance. Your individual needs and circumstances must be taken into account if a blend of this nature is going to work safely. You need to see a professional aromatherapist.

I'm under a great deal of stress right now and feeling overtired, but my partner is asking for sex all the time! Is there anything I can use for her (I'm quite happy to give her a short massage) that will reduce her libido just for a short while so I can get some sleep?

It sounds like you could both do with a bit of support here. Yes, there are essential oils that are 'anaphrodisiacs' – substances which reduce the libido. One of the most effective is marjoram, which is also very handy as it is a good muscle relaxant, a sedative and can clear the respiratory passages too. Try mixing marjoram with lavender and orange – 3 drops each in 15 ml of carrier oil – and using this as a massage blend. There are also a number of essential oils that will help you to relax, get good quality sleep and recover your interest in sex. Try clary sage, vetiver, patchouli or black pepper (black pepper needs to be blended with something like clary sage, geranium or orange if your aim is to aid sleep, as it is a stimulant). See Chapter 10 for more suggestions of oils that help stress and relaxation.

other directions

Aromatherapy and astrology

The idea of using astrology to help determine your choice of essential oils was recently put forward by Patricia Davis in her book, *Astrological Aromatherapy*. (If you want to work with astrology and aromatherapy it is best to gain a thorough knowledge of how astrology works before progressing.)

One of the simplest explanations I have found for astrology is that your natal chart (or natal horoscope) is a representation of how the stars were aligned at the moment of your birth. It functions as a map, showing everything that you came into life intending to work on. It will be very detailed in terms of its descriptions of what influences you, what you are likely to face and what obstacles are most likely to get in your way. To give you the best possible guidance, the astrologer drawing up your chart needs the time (within half an hour), place and date of your birth: without this information, the horoscope will be too vague to be useful.

Most people are familiar with their Sun sign (this is what your daily horoscope in newspapers is based on), and may have an idea of some of the characteristics their Sun sign is supposed to indicate. What you may be less aware of is that the Sun sign represents your most important life lesson: the thing you will work hardest to *be* during your life, or, if you find that you disagree with everything ever written about your particular Sun sign, it may be that your lesson is to accept those characteristics within yourself and how you show them.

However, where things get more complicated is that you really do need to take other factors into consideration when treating an individual with aromatherapy according to their other astrological information:

- the Ascendant – which gives an idea of the face that the person presents to the world (or if you prefer, the mask they wear in public)

- the Moon sign – which indicates emotional personality and can be a key influence where relationships are concerned (as can Venus, if it is about intimate relationships) knowing where Mars is in a person's chart can also be very useful at explaining what has happened should there be problems with their ambitions, their willpower or their drive to succeed (and what it is that they want to succeed at).

If you want to experiment with the ideas behind this method of application, try it on yourself first and consider how closely you are mirroring your own Sun sign from the brief description given below. Remember that you will be expressing your 'key message' in specific ways. For example, a Leo might be here to 'lead' but that can be in all sorts of ways; being the first to try new things, taking charge in a work situation, accepting the situation when it is someone else's turn to be the leader (and not throwing their toys out of the pram), or simply by deciding what is important to them and practising what they preach without being swayed by others (or by shoving their opinions down everyone else's throats).

Sun sign	Key message	Experimental blend
Aries	'I am.' Aries is here to find ways to confirm their personal identity (to decide who they are and what motivates them), to overcome feelings of impatience and to develop the habits necessary to finish what they start.	2 drops each of frankincense, palmarosa rosewood
Taurus	'I have.' Immensely practical (yet artistic), Taurus tends to be very patient and to move as if they are in slow motion. They are here to learn how to let go of their attachments to things or people, to be less stubborn in their thinking and more flexible in their actions.	2 drops each of ginger and grapefruit, 1 of juniper
Gemini	'I think.' The ultimate multi-tasker, Geminis can juggle a range of activities effectively and will be absorbed and interested in all of them. Their task is often to come to a decision about how to focus their attention, and on what. Communication is a key part of their life work – when they aren't communicating their thoughts or feelings, there is something wrong.	3 drops of sandalwood, 1 drop each of cypress and frankincense
Cancer	'I feel.' Feelings run very deep for Cancerians and part of their work is to come to terms with those feelings, to find ways of overcoming any sensations of threat or fear that they feel and to develop an unshakeable sense of security. With that security and self-belief, they can conquer anything.	1 drop of patchouli, 2 drops of vetiver, 3 of rose
Leo	'I lead.' Intense determination, willpower and creativity are what drive Leos forward. Part of their life lesson is to develop an understanding of where they are going (and where they are leading everyone else) as well as to overcome tendencies towards bossiness and attention-seeking behaviour. With no outlet for creative activity, they tend to become depressed.	2 drops of lemongrass, 3 of bergamot, 1 of chamomile
Virgo	'I analyse.' While Virgos' attention to detail can take them very close to perfection in the areas they have chosen to pay attention, their task is to learn to keep their expectations reasonable, to stop seeking perfection in every arena and to slow down on their	2 drops of rose, 1 drop of patchouli, 3 drops of juniper

Sun sign	Key message	Experimental blend
	criticism of self and others before it degenerates into self-loathing.	
Libra	'I balance.' Libras' desire for peaceful compromise makes them great mediators but can also lead to crippling indecision, as well as an overwhelming desire to please others before pleasing themselves. Their task generally involves finding ways of balancing their own needs against those of others and sticking by decisions they have made.	3 drops of ginger, 2 drops of geranium and 1 of frankincense
Scorpio	'I desire.' Emotionally intense and very passionate in their interests, Scorpios are adept at negotiating and cannot be manipulated (although they may try to manipulate others). Part of their lesson is to come to a clear and balanced understanding of their personal power and the depth of their own feelings – learning to let go of occasionally explosive displays of anger in a harmless (and not volcanic) way.	3 drops each of benzoin and palmarosa, 1 drop of jasmine
Sagittarius	'I aspire.' Sagittarians are great at enjoying the journey to any goal they have, sometimes more so than the destination (which can feel like an anticlimax), not least because a thirst for knowledge and experience is being satisfied along the way. A positive and open-minded attitude is their usual state of being, but their personal tasks may involve learning to be less judgmental, especially where they may be expecting too much from life or from others.	3 drops each of neroli and frankincense, 2 drops of cypress
Capricorn	'I use.' A tendency to need to put their knowledge to practical use, anything they do tends to be done well (if not excellently) as they are very focused individuals. Their greatest challenges are to let go of any fear of failure, to rise above depressive states and to learn to 'go with the flow', leaving behind rigid thinking and bossiness.	2 drops each of geranium, black pepper and clary sage
Aquarius	'I know.' Aquarians' focus on the future makes them adept at analysing or predicting trends in whatever area they are interested in. Mentally restless, there is a tendency to rebel against people or situations they feel unable to change. Overcoming the conflicting needs to engage in order to rebel and to disengage in order to remain aloof is part of their personal task.	2 drops each of cedarwood, grapefruit and palmarosa
Pisces	'I believe.' Intuitive, creative and focused on their ideals, Pisceans will occasionally drop everything in order to pursue those ideals, even if the disappearing act causes confusion in friends, families and loved ones. They are extremely good at not facing the reality of any given situation, and benefit enormously if they can learn to overcome this denial of reality and any crippling sense of guilt that might arise thereof.	2 drops each of ginger and rose, 3 drops of juniper

Aromatherapy and Ayurveda

There is a growing interest in the effectiveness of Ayurvedic concepts as a means of choosing and applying essential oils. As with astrology, this works much better if you have a deep understanding of how Ayurveda works.

Ayurveda is based on a five-element theory that is similar in some ways to that of Traditional Chinese Medicine (TCM). Ayurveda involves: Ether (the space where anything can happen), Air (the power to catalyse reactions as oxygen will feed a fire), Fire (the energy to transform), Water (change, the ability to dissolve) and Earth (stability, fixedness). (The five elements of TCM include metal in place of Ether and has significant differences in how the elements are characterised.)

In Ayurveda, the five elements combine in pairs to form three *doshas* or life forces. Each individual is made up of a combination of the three *doshas* – *Vata*, *Pitta* and *Kapha*, although usually, one type will be dominant. Because there is a certain amount of cross-over, some of the essential oils that you might use to treat imbalances in their life force (particularly in their emotional and mental states) will also appear in more than one place.

Dosha type	Signs to look for	Recommended essential oils
Vata	Thin, bird-like (very tall or short, light frame, long fingers), gain weight around the waist, dry skin and brittle nails, variable appetite, restless and active mind, tendency to insomnia	angelica, basil, bergamot, clary sage, eucalyptus, lemon, orange, pine, tangerine, cardamon, chamomile, coriander, fennel, lavender, nutmeg, rosewood, clove, frankincense, ginger, myrrh, rose
Vata–Pitta	Combining features of both Vata and Pitta: talkative, very strong intellectually, occasionally problems with addiction	rose, vetiver, bergamot, lemon, orange, pine, tangerine, cardamon, chamomile, coriander, fennel, lavender, nutmeg, rosewood, clove, frankincense, ginger, lemongrass, clary sage, sandalwood
Pitta–Vata	Quick-moving, physically strong, insecure when stressed, excellent memories	rose, vetiver, bergamot, lemon, orange, pine, tangerine, chamomile, coriander, fennel, lavender, nutmeg, rosewood, clove, frankincense, ginger, lemongrass, clary sage, sandalwood, patchouli, neroli
Pitta	Medium frame, weight gain is deposited evenly, sunburns easily, light eyes, oily skin, often thirsty, competitive, aggressive, jealous and angry when stressed, passionate, focused	bergamot, lemon, lemongrass, lime, orange, clary sage, coriander, fennel, peppermint, jasmine, myrrh, rose, sandalwood, valerian, vetiver

Dosha type	Signs to look for	Recommended essential oils
Pitta–Kapha	Intense, yet physically stable and very strong, plenty of energy and endurance, very strong immune system	bergamot, lemon, lemongrass, lime, orange, clary sage, coriander, fennel, peppermint, jasmine, myrrh, rose, sandalwood, valerian, vetiver
Kapha–Pitta	Kapha shape, but more fat (evenly distributed), slow moving, relaxed, not motivated to exercise (although they are very strong and able when they do work out)	lemon, lemongrass, orange, clary sage, coriander, fennel, peppermint, jasmine, myrrh, rose, sandalwood, valerian, basil, pine, black pepper, chamomile, cinnamon, ginger, juniper, peppermint, rosemary, cardamom, clove, cypress, cedarwood, myrrh, neroli, nutmeg, rose, sandalwood,
Kapha	Large body, heavy bones, square-shaped hands and fingers, weight gain is to hips and thighs, large even teeth, thick skin, tendency to chest infections, laid-back approach to life	basil, lemon, lemongrass, niaouli, orange, pine, black pepper, chamomile, cinnamon, clary sage, coriander, ginger, juniper, peppermint, rosemary, cardamon, clove, cypress, cedarwood, myrrh, neroli, nutmeg, rose, sandalwood, valerian
Kapha–Vata	Slow moving, even tempered, relaxed, very good stamina, hate the cold, chest infections, but otherwise athletic	basil, lemon, lemongrass, niaouli, orange, pine, black pepper, chamomile, cinnamon, clary sage, coriander, ginger, juniper, peppermint, rosemary, cardamon, clove, cypress, cedarwood, myrrh, neroli, nutmeg, rose, sandalwood, valerian, eucalyptus, tangerine, chamomile, fennel, lavender, rosewood, frankincense, myrrh
Vata–Kapha	Contradictory – thin frame, easy-going, even-tempered under stress, very efficient, but will procrastinate	basil, lemon, lemongrass, niaouli, orange, pine, black pepper, cinnamon, clary sage, coriander, ginger, juniper, peppermint, rosemary, cardamom, clove, cypress, cedarwood, myrrh, neroli, nutmeg, rose, sandalwood, valerian, angelica, basil, bergamot, eucalyptus, lemon, tangerine, chamomile, fennel, lavender, rosewood, frankincense

135

Learning how to work with the Ayurvedic principles can take a long time and will involve a lot of learning. You can experiment initially with this in a number of ways. First, you need to work out what your *dosha* type is, especially if it is not easily recognisable from the table given here. Most of the information involved in recognising *dosha* types require you to complete detailed questionnaires, which will include everything from your physical appearance to the frequency and consistency of your bowel movements; where and how you tend to get physical disorders; your moods; your response to stress and how you handle your emotions. Second, treating imbalances in the different *doshas* will involve more than just working with aromatherapy –

you may need to branch into using herbal remedies, altering exercise and eating habits and much more. Where aromatherapy is concerned, you may want to try using the essential oils recommended for the particular *dosha* type you have identified. Use slightly more of the essential oils which you notice are relevant for the *dosha* type you wish to strengthen. So, for example if you know you are a *Kapha–Vata* type, are currently suffering with chest infections and you also know that you have taken the concept of 'procrastination' to its fullest expression (or you would if you could work up the energy), you could try ginger (2 drops), cardamon (3 drops) and cedarwood (3 drops), in 20 ml of carrier oil.

where to go from here

If you have enjoyed this book, learned something and had fun in the process, then it has been a success. That may be as far as you want to take it. But you may want to learn more. You have a wide variety of options at this point:

- Find a short course which will enhance your understanding of a particular aspect of aromatherapy or which will cover different essential oils.

- Carry on and get a professional qualification in aromatherapy.

- Get a professional qualification in another therapy.

Short courses in aromatherapy

Short courses in aromatherapy are on offer all the time, and your local colleges, both public and private, will have at least one (if not several) kinds of introductory courses available. You may find introductory level aromatherapy courses on aromatherapy facials, hand and foot care, aromatherapy for mothers and babies, for partners, for stress relief, for detoxification or aromatherapy and the zodiac – and many others.

Professional aromatherapy courses

Professional courses in aromatherapy are widely available. The majority are offered in Further Education colleges, some higher education colleges (and as part of foundation or undergraduate degree programmes in some universities), community education colleges and in a large number of private colleges. It can be very difficult to choose between the learning establishments as well as the different courses, so take your time making your decision about how you want to learn and where. You may find it helpful to consider the following questions.

When are you are able to attend classes?

Most of the courses available through FE colleges are part-time courses, scheduled to take place once or twice a week. You would have to set aside at least one evening (or part of a day) per week, usually for about one academic year. Private colleges tend to offer more flexibility in their timing – courses will be available on weekends or as a module where you would take an intensive course of training prior to sitting your exams.

Do you want a degree or a vocational course?

Foundation Degree and Honours Degree courses in complementary therapies are available through some FE colleges and some of the more proactive universities. If you are considering a degree course, you will need to ask how much practical work is involved in the degree and whether the professional therapeutic qualifications are embedded in the course. Degree courses will offer you a fascinating and strongly theoretical basis to your understanding of how aromatherapy as well as a number of other therapeutic disciplines work. They do not always prepare you to practise on members of the public. Sometimes it is advisable to go on to degree courses once you have gained your professional qualifications.

Where is the college located and how easy is it for me to get there?

You may want to visit the college you will be learning at to see how easy it is to get to, as well as to view the training rooms you will be having your classes in. This will often give you a good idea about the facilities the tutor will

be using as well as the variety of resources they will have access to in order to enhance your learning experience.

How much does it cost?

Many of the courses run through FE colleges and community education are cheaper than those run through higher education and private colleges. This is because the government often funds part of the course in order to make it more accessible and inviting to new students (especially if it leads to a qualification). However, there are distinct benefits to learning through a private college. Apart from the flexibility in timing, the quality of teaching tends to be good (partly because they pay their tutors more), you are likely to get more personal attention in class and there is often a more informal learning environment. The private colleges may also have a reputation for excellence or additional learning features which would justify the higher fees.

Will my learning support needs be met?

If you have special educational needs or feel you would benefit from additional support while you are learning, you must raise this with the college you are interested in. All the colleges are required to have policies about how they address special learning needs, and you will want to check that you are happy with the support that you have been promised.

How will I be assessed?

Although all professional aromatherapy qualifications in Britain are set at the equivalent of NVQ level 3, there are differences in the methods of assessment used. For example, with certain examining boards, all practical assessment is carried out by your tutor and checked by another tutor in the college. Other examining boards have an external practical examiner who visits the college at the end of the course and watches you (and your classmates) carry out a treatment under timed conditions as well as asking you specific questions related to your work. Theory assessment, meanwhile, can involve coursework, oral examinations, college-set examinations or externally-set and marked examinations, or a combination of the above. These exams can be multiple-choice, short answer, or essay questions, depending on the examining board. Even if you are fearful of examinations, remember that your tutor and the college are there to support you and prepare you for your final assessments. If your fear of examinations is particularly debilitating, there are courses that have no external examinations at all. However, there are situations where exams are infinitely preferable to excessive amounts of coursework.

Are there any added extras?

These are most frequently seen in the private colleges, where your course may have a widely recognised professional qualification embedded within it, but you would be expected to learn additional techniques or theory above and beyond the requirements of the qualification offered. For example, you may choose a course which also includes specialist massage techniques or applications, introductory material from another discipline (such as Traditional Chinese Medicine) and/or specialist information on subjects such as nutrition, counselling, or spiritual healing.

How wide is the range of essential oils covered?

A number of the private colleges offer aromatherapy training which goes beyond the standard number of essential oils covered. For a professional level course, you should be receiving detailed coverage of at least forty essential oils. Where sixty essential oils (or more) are covered, you will be at a distinct advantage, especially if the detailed knowledge of the application of the essential oils is your main reason for undertaking the course.

Is it possible to get accreditation of prior learning?

Each college and examination board will have set different criteria about what they recognise as prior learning that would exempt you from particular sections of the course. For example, whatever course you choose to take, you will be expected to pass examinations in anatomy and physiology, and massage.

How long will it take me to qualify?

Aromatherapy training involves qualifying in anatomy and physiology, and massage, as well as undertaking classes in the biology and application of essential oils. Some colleges insist that you pass your qualifications in these subjects before you start aromatherapy training. Although it is possible to do the courses at the same time, the amount of work and study involved can be quite extensive (especially if case studies are a requirement). Expect to take at least one year to qualify as a therapist (this assumes you will be doing nothing else that year). If the option exists, you may want to consider spreading your learning out over two academic years.

Which professional associations recognise the course?

Taking a course in aromatherapy with the intent to practise professionally would be a waste of time if, after completing your course, you could not get insurance to practise because the course isn't recognised by one of the governing bodies. If you are already aware of and interested in a professional association that you intend to join, visit their website or ask for details about the schools they recommend before making your final decision.

Getting a professional qualification in another therapy

Aromatherapy isn't for everyone. You may decide you would prefer another therapy. For example, you may want to consider:

- a therapy where your client remains clothed – try reflexology, shiatsu, or Indian head massage

- something that specialises in aesthetic applications – for example, beauty therapy

- a therapy that concentrates on the mind and emotions – counselling, life coaching, art or music therapy, or perhaps flower remedies

- an approach that involves working with the flow of life force or universal energy and doesn't necessarily involve touching someone – for example, reiki or spiritual healing

- a more academic route with a highly regarded career path within the National Health Service. Although aromatherapy is widely accepted within a variety of disciplines, it is not yet fully recognised within the NHS. Physiotherapy, osteopathy, chiropractic and acupuncture are now all recognised. Training for these careers starts at degree level and will involve at least three years of learning. Osteopaths, for example, train for five years.

These suggestions are just the beginning of a very long list of disciplines that you may want to consider. Remember, however, that no learning is ever wasted. Enjoy.

Essential oils for mental and emotional support

Essential oil	Sedatives	Stimulants	Euphorics	Aphrodisiacs	Regulators
Cedarwood			●	●	
Benzoin	●		●		●
Bergamot			●		●
Black Pepper		●		●	
Cardamon		●			
Chamomile G	●				
Chamomile R	●				
Clary Sage	●		●	●	
Coriander	●				
Cypress		●			
Eucalyptus		●			
Fennel		●			
Frankincense			●		●
Geranium					●
Ginger		●		●	
Grapefruit		●	●		
Jasmine		●	●	●	
Juniper		●			
Lavender	●				
Lemon		●			
Lemongrass		●			
Marjoram	●			●	
Melissa	●				
Myrrh	●		●		
Neroli	●		●		
Nutmeg		●	●		
Palmarosa		●			
Patchouli				●	
Peppermint		●			
Rosemary		●			
Rose otto			●	●	●
Rosewood	●				
Sandalwood	●			●	
Tea Tree		●			
Valerian	●				
Vetiver	●		●		
Yarrow	●				
Ylang Ylang			●	●	●

FAQs: About progressing with aromatherapy

How do I find out about other essential oils once I've finished my course?

When you start to investigate new essential oils, you need to work in the following ways:

1. First, do a smell test (see Chapter 2) and really concentrate (and note down) how the essential oil makes you feel, both physically and emotionally.

2. Ask the supplier for more information – most essential oil suppliers are in the business because they too have an abiding passion for the essential oils. If they are selling it, they will have information on what it is used for in herbal medicine, as well as interesting ideas about how it has been used in perfumery or in the manufacture of food.

3. Search the internet for references about the oil's use in aromatherapy and particularly for any contraindications.

4. Err on the side of caution. Don't apply it to anyone's skin unless you have first tried vaporising it yourself (and see how you feel), read the instructions or guidelines offered by the suppliers and patch tested it on yourself. Start with it at a very low dilution – no more than 1 or 2 drops in 20 ml of carrier oil.

5. Do a post-graduate course – short courses designed for practising therapists are widely available and are usually advertised via the websites and journals of the various aromatherapy governing bodies.

I heard that once you qualify as an aromatherapist you have to keep going back to study every year. Is this true?

Yes, although this does not only apply to aromatherapy. Most complementary therapists are expected to undergo a certain amount of 'continuing professional development' (CPD) once they are fully qualified. The extent of this depends on the requirements laid down by their governing bodies. It is usually measured as a minimum number of hours of training every year. Post-graduate seminars and workshops will meet these training requirements and some of the governing bodies also recognise time spent reading journals, researching material or writing case studies for publication.

Useful resources

Aromatherapy pre-blended products and essential oils

www.circaroma.co.uk

Essentially Oils
8–19 Mount Farm
Junction Road
Churchill
Chipping Norton OX7 6NP
01608 659544
www.essentiallyoils.com

Tisserand Aromatherapy Products
3 Newtown Road
Hove
Brighton BN3 7BA
www.tisserand.com

Fragrant Earth
Glastonbury
Somerset BA6 9EW
www.fragrant-earth.co.uk

Phytobotanica UK Ltd
Greens Barn
Mill House Plant Farm
Greens Lane
Lydiate
Merseyside
L31 4HZ
01695 420853
www.phytobotanica.com

Quinessence Aromatherapy
Forest Court
Linden Way
Coalville
Leicester LE67 3JY
01530 838358
www.quinessence.com

Finding an aromatherapy course

www.itecworld.co.uk
www.vtct.co.uk
www.ifpa.org.uk
www.hotcourses.com

Essential reading

Battaglia, S. (2003) *The Complete Guide to Aromatherapy* (2nd edn.), International Centre of Holistic Aromatherapy,
Mojay, G. (1996) *Aromatherapy for Healing the Spirit*, Hodder and Stoughton
Dr Light Miller & Dr Bryan Miller, *Ayurveda and Aromatherapy: The Earth Essential Guide to Ancient Wisdom and Modern Healing*, Lotus Press (1995)
Davis, P. (2002) *Astrological Aromatherapy*, C W Daniel

Books by the author

The Aromatherapy Kitchen, Search Press (2000)
Business Practice for Therapists, Hodder and Stoughton (2002)
Massage in Essence, Hodder and Stoughton (2006)
Learn to Sleep, Parragon (2004)
Learn to Relax, Parragon (2004)

Finding an aromatherapist

www.embodyforyou.co.uk
www.ifpa.org.uk

Buying protective clothing

www.dkprofashion.com
www.vitalitywear.co.uk
www.salonsdirect.com

Buying a massage couch

The following all offer standard and professional massage couches at mid-range prices:

- Beautelle
  www.beautelle.co.uk
- Marshcouch

  14 Robinsfield
  Hemel Hempstead HP1 1RW
  01442 263199
  www.marshcouch.com
- New Concept

  www.new-concept.co.uk
- The Massage Table Store

  01454 261900/020 8983 9800
  www.mts4u.com

glossary

Achilles tendon: the tendon that connects the gastrocnemius (calf muscle) to the calcaneus (heel bone).

Acne rosacea: a variety of acne that usually occurs in the late twenties or early thirties. Symptoms include broken capillaries on the cheek, nose and forehead, a tendency to blush easily and a persistent redness to the skin, even if pimples are not visible on the surface.

Acne vulgaris: more commonly regarded as teenage acne, though not exclusive to the young. Symptoms include inflamed pus-filled lesions that can occur anywhere on the body, but appear most frequently on the face, neck, back and chest.

Allergen: a substance that triggers an allergic reaction.

Allergy: a hypersensitive reaction to the presence of a substance such as pollen, dustmites, or certain chemicals or foods. Usually appears either as hay fever-like symptoms (including sneezing), or inflammation of the skin or gut, sometimes accompanied by itchy skin or the appearance of hives. In very serious conditions, anaphylactic shock can develop, where the bronchial tubes and/or throat can swell shut – potentially life threatening.

Alzheimer's disease: disabling dementia, where the person loses the ability to reason and to care for themselves. In severe cases, there can be episodes of hallucination, violent changes of mood and paranoia.

Amenorrhoea: abnormal failure to menstruate.

Analgesic: painkiller.

Anaphrodisiac: reduces sexual desire.

Antihistamine: reduces the amounts of histamine found in the blood or body tissues at any one time. (Histamine is a substance involved in developing inflammation and other aspects of the immune response).

Anti-inflammatory: reduces inflammation.

Antiseptic: kills bacteria (on the skin).

Aphrodisiac: encourages sexual desire.

Arthritis: pain, stiffness, swelling (or inflammation) of the joints.

Ascending colon: The first portion of the colon (or large intestine). It starts at the ileocoecal valve and continues until it reaches the hepatic flexure beneath the liver.

Asthma: respiratory condition that involves chronic inflammation of the airways and an oversensitivity to certain substances. An attack is triggered when the person comes into contact with a stimulus to which they are sensitive. The airways inflame and excessive mucus builds up in the airways which may become obstructed, making breathing very difficult.

Athlete's foot: a fungal infection of the feet, usually found under and around the toes. It is made worse by poor hygiene, not drying the feet properly and wearing shoes that do not allow appropriate air circulation.

Autonomic nervous system: the section of the nervous system responsible for the automatic functioning of the body. It governs actions such as choking, sneezing, coughing, hiccupping, appetite, and the sleep/wake cycle.

145

Axial: area directly underneath the arms (armpits).

Ayurvedic: a system of medical and health beliefs which originated in India and whose practice is based on an understanding of the physical/emotional/energetic body type (or dosha) of the individual.

Bronchitis: inflammation of the bronchial tubes.

Carpals: the bones of the wrist.

Carrier oil: a general term used to describe the vegetable oils in which essential oils are blended in order to spread them evenly over the body.

Catarrh: phlegm or mucus that is expelled from the lungs or pharynx.

Chemoreceptors: nerve endings, usually (with respect to the study of aromatherapy) found in the nose, which register the presence of specific chemicals.

Cirrhosis: a disorder of the liver, usually brought on by excessive alcohol consumption. The liver becomes scarred and is unable to function properly as a result of the presence of too many toxins.

Cold sores: ulcerative sores that usually appear in and around the mouth. They arise as a result of the presence of the herpes zoster virus and recur if the person is under a great deal of stress or their immune system is weak.

Colic: digestion disorder common to infants that causes excessive (and painful) wind. Usually disappears after the age of three months.

Constipation: condition wherein the person is unable to pass a stool. Made worse for poor dietary habits (not enough fruit, vegetables and water).

Contraindication: a reason not to treat. The practitioner may need the permission or advice of another practitioner (for example, a medical practitioner) before treating; it may be best to proceed only with certain provisos; or it may be best to avoid treatment.

Cubital crease: inner crease of the elbow.

Cystitis: inflammation of the bladder.

Cytophylactic: encourages healthy skin repair.

Deltoids: muscles lying over the shoulder that help to raise the arm.

Dermatitis: inflammation of the dermis in the skin.

Descending colon: the third portion of the colon (or large intestine). This starts on the left hand side at the splenic flexure (below the spleen) and goes to the sigmoid flexure (just inside the left hip).

Diaphragm: flat, dome-shaped muscle that separates the thoracic cavity (the rib cage and its contents) from the abdominal cavity.

Diastole: the relaxation phase of the heart – when the heart's chambers (ventricles) fill with blood.

Distillation: in aromatherapy, this refers to the process where boiling water or steam is passed through plant material in order to extract the essential oils.

Diuretic: reduces water retention.

Dosha: the body type as described in ayurvedic medicine. Involves an understanding of the physical as well as emotional and energetic principles.

Dysmenorrhoea: painful periods.

Eczema: skin disorder. Symptoms include an allergic-style response to a substance that has either been exposed to the skin or has been eaten. Often made worse by stress. Usually results in weeping (or bleeding) sores that are intensely itchy.

Effleurage: flowing massage stroke, used before and after all deeper strokes. Deeply relaxing, it can also boost the circulation.

Emmenagogue: a substance that encourages menstruation.

Endometriosis: painful condition in which the endometrial tissue lining the uterus migrates outside the uterus to attach itself to other abdominal organs. As it responds to hormones, it will continue to grow and shed with each menstrual period, resulting in severe bloating, internal bleeding and sometimes difficulty in conceiving.

Enfleurage: method of essential oil extraction where flowers are placed in the chosen carrier oil and left in the sunlight until the essential oils have permeated the carrier oil.

Epilepsy: Condition marked by sudden recurrent episodes of sensory disturbance, loss of consciousness or convulsions. Occurs as a result of abnormal electrical activity in the brain. May develop as a result of genetic inheritance, a blow to the head, infection, high fever, or tumour.

Episiotomy: when the perineal tissues are cut during labour in order to allow the baby to pass out of the mother faster and/or more easily.

Erector spinae: a group of muscles that extend all the way along the spine, helping to keep the back erect and control movement when bending forward.

Essential oil: plant extract, usually obtained by distillation, which is both fragrant and highly volatile. Used in aromatherapy and perfumery, and the cosmetics, food and pharmaceutical industries.

Euphoric: a substance that lifts the mind and spirits, inducing feelings of well-being.

Exfoliate: to scrub and/or remove dead skin cells from the surface of the skin.

Feng shui: ancient Chinese system of laws considered to govern spatial arrangement in relation to the flow of energy.

Fibroids: a growth of tissues, usually found in or around the uterus.

Five element theory: concept found in both Ayurvedic and Traditional Chinese Medicine (TCM). Both disciplines state that all life force is made up of five distinct types of energy. In the Ayurvedic tradition the five elements are Wind, Water, Fire, Earth and Ether. In Chinese medicine they are Fire, Earth, Metal, Water and Wood.

Frontal lobe: the anterior (front) portion of the cerebrum at the top of the brain.

Fungal infections: range of yeast overgrowths found in or on the body. The most common relate to overgrowths of a fungus called *Candida albicans* and include athlete's foot and vaginal, oral and penile thrush.

Gastrocnemius: main calf muscle (gives the top of the calf its characteristic bulging shape); involved in flexing the foot and pointing the toes.

Gingivitis: inflammation of the gums.

Gluteals: the large muscles covering the hips and giving shape to the bottom.

Haemorrhoids: varicose veins of the anus.

Hamstrings: a group of three muscles at the back of the thigh: the semimembranosus, semitendinosus and biceps femoris.

Heart failure: where the heart is failing to pump. Sometimes called congestive heart failure. This can be a result of a number of conditions including long-term high blood pressure, coronary artery disease and valve disorders, or following heart attacks.

Heart palpitations: when the heart can be felt to be beating rapidly or erratically.

Heartburn: acid reflux – acid from the stomach overflows into the oesophagus, usually as a result of pressure from below (if the subject has overeaten, recently gained a lot of weight or is pregnant).

Holistic: something which takes into account a person's physical, mental, emotional, spiritual and environmental circumstances to provide a treatment or product that is appropriate for the individual.

Hormonally-sensitive skin: skin that is prone to blemishes as a result of changes in the menstural cycle or in testosterone levels.

Hydrolats: the water-based by-product of the distillation of essential oils.

Hypertension: high blood pressure (usually, above 175/100).

Hyperthyroidism: when the thyroid produces excessive amounts of its hormones (including thyroxine). Common symptoms are sudden weight loss, excessive sweating, heart palpitations, and the eyes appear to protrude.

Hypotension: low blood pressure (usually, below 100/70).

Hypothalamus: section of the brain involved in maintaining homeostasis (steady conditions) within the body. It controls the autonomic nervous system and the endocrine system (because it controls the action of the pituitary gland which governs the endocrine system), and regulates emotions, eating, drinking and appetites, body temperature and sleep/wake cycles.

Idiosyncratic reaction: a personal and unusual reaction to a substance (in aromatherapy, to an essential oil).

Impetigo: bacterial skin infection common in children that is very itchy.

Irritable bowel syndrome (IBS): Painful and frequent muscle spasms of the gut, accompanied by inflammation and often over-sensitive reactions to food. Common symptoms are alternating constipation and diarrhoea.

Kinesiology: the study of the mechanics of body movements.

Kneading: invigorating massage stroke applied to the body's fleshy areas, where muscles are manipulated in a rhythmic, rolling action, from one hand to the other. Helps break down fatty deposits and eliminate waste products at a deeper level.

Knuckling: deep massage movement where the knuckles of the therapist's hands press and rotate over large areas of muscle. Stimulating; increases circulation.

Lateral: the outer edge.

Levator scapulae: muscle in the neck that helps to raise the shoulder blades.

Ligaments: the inflexible tissues which attach bones to other bones and help to stabilise joints.

Limbic system: sometimes referred to as the emotional brain, this is found deep within the centre of the brain and governs all emotional

behaviour including responses to pleasure, pain, anger, affection and so on.

Lymph: plasma (the liquid part of blood) which has escaped from the blood vessels in order to bathe surrounding tissues in nutrients. Lymph vessels help to transport lymph back to the blood vessels.

Lymphatic congestion: where lymph pools in specific areas of the body. (Also known as oedema.)

Masseter: muscle of the face that helps to close the jaw.

Medial: inner (or middle) section.

Melatonin: a hormone involved in regulating the sleep/wake cycle that requires adjustment where there is jet lag.

Menarche: the onset of puberty in girls.

Menopause: the ending of the menstrual phase of a woman's life. Usually occurs between the ages of 45 and 50 and may be accompanied by symptoms such as hot flushes.

Metacarpals: five bones in the palm of the hand.

Metatarsals: five bones in the foot. They lie between the tarsals (ankle bones) and the phalanges (bones of the toes).

Mitral cells: cells which help to concentrate or amplify fragrances so they can be identified by the olfactory nerve.

Mucus membrane: mucus-producing layer found throughout the body (most noticeably in the nasal and respiratory passages, the gastrointestinal tract and in the vagina). Mucus membranes are an important part of the body's immune response as they protect the body tissues from foreign particles that could cause disease.

Myalgic encephalomyelitis (ME): chronic fatigue syndrome – a post-viral condition where pain and fatigue slow down the rate of recovery.

Neuralgia: nerve pain.

Neurotransmitter: a chemical involved in the transmission of nerve messages.

Occipital bone: bone at the base of the skull.

Oedema: an excess of watery fluid in the cavities or tissues of the body.

Oestrogen: hormone produced by the ovaries that is linked to the development of fertile eggs in women and the development of female secondary sexual characteristics (development of breasts, axial and pubic hair, onset of menstruation and the control of the menstrual cycle).

Olfaction: the sense of smell.

Olfactory adaptation: a phenomena whereby you adapt to a fragrance and cease to notice it.

Oligomenorrhoea: irregular periods.

Orbicularis oris: the circular muscle around the eye which forms the eyelids.

Osteoarthritis: pain, stiffness and swelling of the joints as a result of overuse.

Osteoporosis: a condition of the bones where they become brittle and fragile as a result of a loss of calcium. Most common in older people, although it can develop in younger people, especially in women who cease to menstruate for months or years at a time (perhaps as a result of sudden weight loss, over-exercising or illness). Linked to poor eating habits, not enough exercise, smoking and alcohol intake.

Parkinson's disease: progressive disease of the brain and nervous system marked by involuntary skeletal muscle contractions (tremors), muscle rigidity and slow, imprecise movements.

Patch testing: method you can use to ensure that clients are not likely to react negatively to any blend of essential oils that you use. Essential oils (or carrier oils) can be tested on a small area of skin to ensure there is no adverse reaction prior to being used in a massage.

Pectorals: the group of muscles which cover the ribcage.

Percussion: rapid massage movements used in Swedish, holistic and therapeutic massage, which draw the circulation towards the skin. Revitalising and toning in effect; often used near the end of a massage to increase alertness and vitality. Percussive strokes include cupping (using the hands in a cup shape), hacking (using the sides of the hands), and pummelling (using the underside of the fists).

Perineum: area of muscle between the anus and the scrotum or vulva.

Petrissage: deep pressure massage strokes, applied after preparation with effleurage and kneading, which pushes the tissue towards the bone. Helps to break down waste products in the muscles by pressing of muscles into the bones underlying them . Can be used as a firm, releasing stretch.

Phlebitis: inflammation of the blood vessels (usually of the veins).

Photosensitisation: refers to adverse reaction (usually itching or burning sensation) that some essential oils may produce in the skin in the presence of sunlight.

Piriformis: muscle deep beneath the gluteals which joins the sacrum to the head of the femur and is usually involved in problems with sciatica.

Polycystic ovarian syndrome (PCOS): a condition in which multiple cysts grow on the ovaries. The cysts limit the development of eggs or the release of oestrogen, resulting in a range of symptoms including sudden weight gain, growth of male pattern hair, lack of periods, loss of fertility and potentially, early menopause.

Popliteal: refers to the region of the hollow at the back of the knee, where the lymph nodes are located.

Postnatal depression: depressive state that develops in some women after the birth of a child. Symptoms vary greatly.

Post-viral fatigue: muscle pain and fatigue which develop after exposure to a virus. Recovery is often prolonged.

Pre-eclampsia: dangerous condition found in pregnant women which involves very high blood pressure and where blood supply to the infant can be reduced.

Progesterone: hormone produced by the ovaries which ensures that the uterus is prepared for implantation of a fertilised ovum. High levels of progesterone are linked to pre-menstrual symptoms.

Prone: lying face down.

Psoriasis: inflammatory skin condition where certain skin cells divide faster and move more quickly to the surface of the skin than they would normally do. They form flaky, silvery scales on the surface of the skin (usually in the scalp, the knees or the elbows) over reddened areas.

Restless leg syndrome: unpleasant sensation in the legs, relieved by movement. Leads to constant movement during the day and often to insomnia at night.

Rheumatoid arthritis: pain, stiffness and swelling of the joints as a result of an autoimmune reaction (where the body starts to attack itself). Commoner in women, the average age at which it appears is 35 years.

Rhinitis: inflammation of the mucus membranes in the nasal passages which results in an overproduction of mucus.

Rhomboid: muscle lying between the scapula (shoulder blade) and the spine which pulls the scapula towards the spine.

Ringworm: a fungal infection which results in a distinctive circular pattern on the skin.

Rotator cuff muscles: a group of muscles involved in helping the shoulder to rotate, including the supraspinatus, infraspinatus, teres minor, teres major and subscapularis.

Sacrum: flat bone found at the base of the spine.

Sciatica: pain associated with the sciatic nerve which travels down the back of the leg from the hip joint to the heel. Pain can be debilitating.

Seasonal affective disorder (SAD): depressive condition linked to the amount of sunlight the person is exposed to (the condition is worsened in cold, dark weather).

Sebum: oily substance produced by the skin which provides weatherproofing and protection against drying out and some types of infection.

Senile dementia: see Alzheimer's disease.

Sensitisation: where a substance, in this case an essential oil, encourages an adverse skin reaction to develop.

Sinusitis: inflammation of the sinuses.

Sleep apnoea: a condition in which the person ceases to breath for short periods during sleep. Usually the muscles around the throat relax, collapsing the trachea and cutting off the oxygen supply. The person may wake up suddenly (or partially wake) in order to start breathing again. Usually accompanied by noticeable snoring. Most often the person feels that they do not get good quality sleep (as they keep waking up).

Soleus: muscle found in the posterior calf.

Supine: lying face up.

Supraspinatus: muscle found at the top of the shoulder blade.

Synergistic blend/synergy: a blend where the effect of the combination of essential oils is greater if used separately.

Systole: the contraction phase of the heartbeat, when the heart contracts and pushes blood out into the arteries.

Tapotement: range of vibratory movements used in Swedish, holistic and therapeutic massage. Shakes and loosens specific muscles by vibrating the fingers against a fleshy area. Has a stimulating effect.

Thalamus: inner portion of the brain involved in the acquisition and retention of knowledge. It also relays sensory impulses from the cerebrum to the spinal cord and other parts of the brain.

Thread veins: tiny, visible blood vessels near the surface of the skin.

Thrombosis: local coagulation or clotting of the blood.

Thrush: painful and itchy yeast infection, usually found in the mouth, vagina or penis.

TMJ: the temporal-mandibular joint (where the jaw attaches to the skull, just in front of the ears).Teeth- grinding may result in pain in this area.

Transverse colon: section of the colon which runs across the body from the hepatic flexure to splenic flexure (right to left).

Trapezius: major muscle of the upper back.

Varicose veins: condition of the veins which occurs when blood pools in the area and causes the walls of the veins to distend.

Verucca: highly infectious wart found on the base (plantar surface) of the foot.

Volatility: a measure of the ability of a compound, such as an essential oil, to react to other compounds and particularly to exposure to air. More volatile compounds will react faster.

Wart: small, hard benign growth on the skin.

Zygomaticus: muscle lying over the cheekbone, involved in smiling.

index

GUILDFORD **college**

Learning Resource Centre

Please return on or before the last date shown.
No further issues or renewals if any items are overdue.

Class: 615.3219 JEN

Title: Aromatherapy in Essence

Author: Jenkins, Nicola